Pat Precin, MS, OTR
Editor

Surviving 9/11: Impact and Experiences of Occupational Therapy Practitioners

Surviving 9/11: Impact and Experiences of Occupational Therapy Practitioners has been co-published simultaneously as *Occupational Therapy in Mental Health*, Volume 19, Numbers 3/4 2003.

Pre-publication REVIEWS, COMMENTARIES, EVALUATIONS . . .

"This book will serve not only as AN EXCELLENT TRAINING TOOL for anyone whose work may include helping others in a disaster, but readers from all walks of life will be moved by its INSIGHTFUL AND STIRRING accounts of people acting in the face of unthinkable events."

Scott A. Bennett, MSEd
Founder, click4careercoaching.com

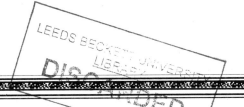

More pre-publication
REVIEWS, COMMENTARIES, EVALUATIONS . . .

"This book IMPARTS KNOWLEDGE ABOUT DISASTER MENTAL HEALTH COUNSELING TECHNIQUES, PTSD, SPIRITUALITY, COPING, AND MOST IMPORTANTLY THE HUMAN BOND THAT IS CREATED BY THE OT CLINICIAN AND HER CLIENTS. The book's authors show what outstanding clinicians they are, whether the people they are helping are patients, students, neighbors, colleagues, friends, or strangers. As a person who lives three blocks from ground zero, 9/11 is a real felt event. 9/11 forever changed our world, our country, my city, and my life. Reading this book brought back the memories of that time, both the trauma and the community pride associated with recovery from an unthinkable crisis."

Suzanne White, OTR, MA
Clinical Assistant Professor,
OT Program,
SUNY Downstate Medical Center

"I RECOMMEND THIS BOOK to anyone who experienced the pain of 9/11–to whatever degree. IT SHOWS THE TRUE MEANING OF OCCUPATION AND PARTICIPATION FOLLOWING TRAGEDY by telling the stories of survivors, rescuers, OT practitioners, and volunteers. The many compelling stories in this book convey the powerful message that individuals and communities recover from such monumental loss 'through engagement, [in] one meaningful activity at a time.' This book is a healing work. As a family member of a victim of 9/11, I read each chapter with my tissues in hand and felt comforted by the shared stories. We have so much to learn from the experiences of others in the face of such an unimaginable tragedy, and how engagement and participation can help us all heal."

Barbara L. Kornblau, JD, OT/L, FAOTA, DAAPM, CCM
President, American Occupational
Therapy Association,
Professor, Occupational Therapy,
Law & Public Health,
Nova Southeastern University

The Haworth Press, Inc.

Surviving 9/11:
Impact and Experiences
of Occupational Therapy
Practitioners

Surviving 9/11: Impact and Experiences of Occupational Therapy Practitioners has been co-published simultaneously as *Occupational Therapy in Mental Health*, Volume 19, Numbers 3/4 2003.

Occupational Therapy in Mental Health Monographic "Separates"

Below is a list of "separates," which in serials librarianship means a special issue simultaneously published as a special journal issue or double-issue _and_ as a "separate" hardbound monograph. (This is a format which we also call a "DocuSerial.")

"Separates" are published because specialized libraries or professionals may wish to purchase a specific thematic issue by itself in a format which can be separately cataloged and shelved, as opposed to purchasing the journal on an on-going basis. Faculty members may also more easily consider a "separate" for classroom adoption.

"Separates" are carefully classified separately with the major book jobbers so that the journal tie-in can be noted on new book order slips to avoid duplicate purchasing.

You may wish to visit Haworth's website at . . .

http://www.HaworthPress.com

. . . to search our online catalog for complete tables of contents of these separates and related publications.

You may also call 1-800-HAWORTH (outside US/Canada: 607-722-5857), or Fax 1-800-895-0582 (outside US/Canada: 607-771-0012), or e-mail at:

docdelivery@haworthpress.com

Surviving 9/11: Impact and Experiences of Occupational Therapy Practitioners, edited by Pat Precin, MS, OTR/L (Vol. 19, No. 3/4 2003). *Analyzes the many roles occupational therapy practitioners played during the tragic events of 9/11; examines new therapeutic practices developed because of the terrorist attacks.*

An Ethnographic Study of Mental Health Treatment and Outcomes: Doing What Works, by Fran Babiss, PhD, OTR/L (Vol. 18, No. 3/4, 2002). *"All mental health clinicians and scholars will find this book INSIGHTFUL AND PROVOCATIVE. This book contains more than a description of three women living with anorexia nervosa; the rich qualitative data captures their pain and their struggles with daily life to survive." (Jim Hinojosa, PhD, OT, FAOTA, Professor and Chair, Department of Occupational Therapy, New York University)*

Recovery and Wellness: Models of Hope and Empowerment for People with Mental Illness, edited by Catana Brown, PhD, OTR/L, FAOTA (Vol. 17, No. 3/4, 2001). *Provides guidelines for incorporating wellness and recovery principles into mental health services using the Recovery Model.*

Domestic Abuse Across the Lifespan: The Role of Occupational Therapy, by Christine A. Helfrich, PhD, OTR/L (Vol. 16, No. 3/4, 2001). *"For those occupational therapists who view themselves as holistic service providers, this book is a must-read. . . . Includes examples, studies, and research results." (Linda T. Learneard, OTR/L, President, Occupational Therapy Consultation and Rehabilitation Services, Inc.)*

Brain Injury and Gender Role Strain: Rebuilding Adult Lifestyles After Injury, by Sharon A. Gutman, PhD, OTR (Vol. 15, No. 3/4, 2000). *"Dr. Gutman has developed an innovative target setting and treatment planning protocol that focuses the therapist on the key areas of concern. I highly recommend this book to therapists who work with clients in the post-acute period of recovery from TBI." (Gordon Muir Giles, MA, Dip COT, OTR, Director of Neurobehavioral Services, Crestwood Behavioral Health, Inc., and Assistant Professor, Samuel Merritt College, Oakland, California)*

New Frontiers in Psychosocial Occupational Therapy, edited by Anne Hiller Scott, PhD, OTR, FAOTA (Vol. 14, No. 1/2, 1998). *"Speaks a clear message about mental health practice in occupational therapy, shattering old visions of practice to insights about empowerment and advocacy." (Sharan L. Schwartzberg, EdD, OTR, FAOTA, Professor and Chair, Boston School of Occupational Therapy, Tufts University)*

Evaluation and Treatment of the Psychogeriatric Patient, edited by Diane Gibson, MS, OTR (Vol. 10, No. 3, 1991). *"Occupational therapists everywhere, learners and sophisticates alike, and in-hospital and out-patient areas as well as home-bound and home-active, would enjoy and profit from this exposition as much as I did."* (American Association of Psychiatric Administrators)

Student Recruitment in Psychosocial Occupational Therapy: Intergenerational Approaches, edited by Susan Haiman (Vol. 10, No. 1, 1990). *"Can serve to enlighten both academics and clinicians as to their roles in attracting students to become practitioners in mental health settings. Each article could well serve as a catalyst for discussion in the classroom or clinic."* (Canadian Journal of Occupational Therapy)

Group Protocols: A Psychosocial Compendium, edited by Susan Haiman (Vol. 9, No. 4, 1990). *"Presents succinct protocols for a wide range of groups that are typically run by activities therapists, vocational counselors, art therapists, and other mental health professionals."* (International Journal of Group Psychotherapy)

Instrument Development in Occupational Therapy, edited by Janet Hawkins Watts and Chestina Brollier (Vol. 8, No. 4, 1989). *Examines content and concurrent validity and development of the Assessment of Occupational Functioning (AOF), and carefully compares the AOF with a similar instrument, the Occupational Case Analysis Interview and Rating Scale (OCAIRS), to discover the similarities and strengths of these instruments.*

Group Process and Structure in Psychosocial Occupational Therapy, edited by Diane Gibson, MS, OTR (Vol. 8, No. 3, 1989). *Highly skilled professionals examine the important concepts of group therapy to help build cohesive, safe groups.*

Treatment of Substance Abuse: Psychosocial Occupational Therapy Approaches, edited by Diane Gibson, MS, OTR (Vol. 8, No. 2, 1989). *A unique overview of contemporary assessment and rehabilitation of alcohol and chemical dependent substance abusers.*

The Development of Standardized Clinical Evaluations in Mental Health, Principal Investigator: Noomi Katz, PhD, OTR; edited by Claudia Kay Allen, MA, OTR, FAOTA; Commentator: Janice P. Burke, MA, OTR, FAOTA (Vol. 8, No. 1, 1988). *"Contains a collection of research-based articles encompassing several evaluations that can be used by occupational therapists practicing in mental health."* (American Journal of Occupational Therapy)

Evaluation and Treatment of Adolescents and Children, edited by Diane Gibson, MS, OTR (Vol. 7, No. 2, 1987). *Experts share research results and practices that have proven successful in helping young people who suffer from psychiatric and medical disorders.*

Treatment of the Chronic Schizophrenic Patient, edited by Diane Gibson, MS, OTR (Vol. 6, No. 2, 1986). *"Reflect[s] creative and fresh concepts of current treatment for the chronically mentally ill. . . . Recommended for the therapist practicing in psychiatry."* (Canadian Journal of Occupational Therapy)

The Evaluation and Treatment of Eating Disorders, edited by Diane Gibson, MS, OTR (Vol. 6, No. 1, 1986). *"A wealth of information. . . . Covers the subject thoroughly. . . . This book, well-conceived and well-written, is recommended not only for clinicians working with clients with anorexia nervosa and bulimia but for all therapists who wish to become acquainted with the subject of eating disorders in general."* (Library Journal)

Philosophical and Historical Roots of Occupational Therapy, edited by Karen Diasio Serrett (Vol. 5, No. 3, 1985). *"Recommended as an easy-to-get-through background read for occupational therapists and for generalists wishing a fuller acquaintance with the backdrop of occupational therapy."* (Rehabilitation Literature)

Short-Term Treatment in Occupational Therapy, edited by Diane Gibson, MS, OTR, and Kathy Kaplan, MS, OTR (Vol. 4, No. 3, 1984). *"Thought provoking and relevant to various issues facing OTs in a short term inpatient psychiatric setting. . . . Very readable . . . concise, well-written, and stimulating."* (Canadian Journal of Occupational Therapy)

SCORE: Solving Community Obstacles and Restoring Employment, by Lynn Wechsler Kramer, MS, OTR (Vol. 4, No. 1, 1984). *"This needed book is an effective instrument for occupational therapists wanting to 'teach employable handicapped how to obtain a job in a competitive*

(labor) market.' Very relevant to professional practice . . . a useful how-to instrument."
(The American Journal of Occupational Therapy)

Occupational Therapy with Borderline Patients, edited by Diane Gibson, MS, OTR (Vol. 3, No. 3, 1983). *"Offers clinicians an opportunity to review current theoretical concepts, management, and design of activity groups for this population. Well written . . . provides good reference lists and well-developed discussions." (The American Journal of Occupational Therapy)*

Psychiatric Occupational Therapy in the Army, edited by LTC Paul D. Ellsworth, MPH, OTR, FAOTA, and Diane Gibson, MS, OTR (Vol. 3, No. 2, 1983). *This unique volume focuses on the historical contributions, current trends, and future directions of army occupational therapists practicing in the military mental health arena.*

Surviving 9/11: Impact and Experiences of Occupational Therapy Practitioners

Pat Precin, MS, OTR/L
Editor

Surviving 9/11: Impact and Experiences of Occupational Therapy Practitioners has been co-published simultaneously as *Occupational Therapy in Mental Health*, Volume 19, Numbers 3/4 2003.

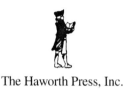

The Haworth Press, Inc.

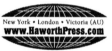

New York • London • Victoria (AU)
www.HaworthPress.com

Surviving 9/11: Impact and Experiences of Occupational Therapy Practitioners has been co-published simultaneously as *Occupational Therapy in Mental Health*™, Volume 19, Numbers 3/4 2003.

Cover design by Lora Wiggins

Library of Congress Cataloging-in-Publication Data

Surviving 9/11 : impact and experiences of occupational therapy practitioners / [edited by] Pat Precin.
     p. ; cm.
"Co-published simultaneously as Occupational therapy in mental health, Volume 19, Numbers 3/4."
Includes bibliographical references and index.
    ISBN 0-7890-2066-1 (hard cover : alk. paper) – ISBN 0-7890-2067-X (soft cover : alk. paper)
    1. Occupational therapy. 2. September 11 Terrorist Attacks, 2001–Psychological aspects. 3. Disaster victims–Mental health. 4. Disasters–Psychological aspects. 5. Crisis intervention (Mental health services)
    [DNLM: 1. Emergencies–psychology–New York City. 2. Disasters–New York City. 3. Occupational Therapy–psychology–New York City. 4. Survival–psychology–New York City. WB 105 S963 2003] I. Title: Surviving nine eleven. II. Precin, Pat.
    RM735.S87 2003
    616.89´165–dc22
                           2003019038

Indexing, Abstracting & Website/Internet Coverage

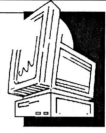

This section provides you with a list of major indexing & abstracting services. That is to say, each service began covering this periodical during the year noted in the right column. Most Websites which are listed below have indicated that they will either post, disseminate, compile, archive, cite or alert their own Website users with research-based content from this work. (This list is as current as the copyright date of this publication.)

(continued)

  * Exact start date to come.

Special Bibliographic Notes related to special journal issues (separates) and indexing/abstracting:

- indexing/abstracting services in this list will also cover material in any "separate" that is co-published simultaneously with Haworth's special thematic journal issue or DocuSerial. Indexing/abstracting usually covers material at the article/chapter level.
- monographic co-editions are intended for either non-subscribers or libraries which intend to purchase a second copy for their circulating collections.
- monographic co-editions are reported to all jobbers/wholesalers/approval plans. The source journal is listed as the "series" to assist the prevention of duplicate purchasing in the same manner utilized for books-in-series.
- to facilitate user/access services all indexing/abstracting services are encouraged to utilize the co-indexing entry note indicated at the bottom of the first page of each article/chapter/contribution.
- this is intended to assist a library user of any reference tool (whether print, electronic, online, or CD-ROM) to locate the monographic version if the library has purchased this version but not a subscription to the source journal.
- individual articles/chapters in any Haworth publication are also available through the Haworth Document Delivery Service (HDDS).

DEDICATION

Dedicated to the heroes of 9/11: victims, survivors and helpers; to the inner strength, courage, and resilience of the human spirit; to life and to the power of the moment.

ABOUT THE EDITOR

Pat Precin, MS, OTR/L, is currently the Managing Director of Pathways to Housing, Inc., a housing-first, consumer-driven organization that provides scattered site apartments and assertive community treatment to chronically homeless individuals with mental illness and substance abuse. She has been the Director of the Brooklyn Bureau of Community Service's P.R.I.D.E. 2000 Program (Personal Roads to Individual Development and Employment), a performance-based Welfare-to-Work initiative that helps disabled public assistance recipients find and retain gainful employment. She has also directed the Occupational, Recreational and Creative Arts Therapy Programs at St. Luke's-Roosevelt Hospital in New York City. She is Adjunct Assistant Professor of Occupational Therapy at LaGuardia Community College and has directly supervised over 100 occupational therapy students in various clinical settings. Having twelve years of clinical experience in the areas of psychosocial occupational therapy and substance abuse, she has authored two additional books on clinical reasoning and dual diagnosis (substance abuse and mental illness), multiple journal articles and grants, as well as performed research studies in these fields. She serves on the Educational Board of the State University of New York Downstate Medical Center's Occupational Therapy Program, and of LaGuardia Community College, on the board of Housing First, Inc., and on the Board of Directors of the Center for Community Integration, Inc. She works actively with the Metropolitan New York State District Occupational Therapy Association (MNYD of NYSOTA) Mental Health Task Force. She has degrees in Biophysics, Psychology, Pre-medicine and Occupational Therapy and is a member of the following national honor fraternities: Tri Beta (biology), Psy Chi (Psychology), and Mu Phi Epsilon (Music). Pat has been a long-term consultant for a consumer-owned and run non-profit organization that guides mental health consumer entrepreneurs through their business ventures. She has spoken at international, national, and state conferences and at colleges and universities. Pat is dedicated to continuous quality improvement and the achievement of measurable outcomes in all of the endeavors above. She has also been a published poet, professional musician, competitive athlete, photographer, and cave diver/explorer.

Surviving 9/11: Impact and Experiences of Occupational Therapy Practitioners

CONTENTS

About the Contributors

Fran Babiss, PhD, OTR/L, is an occupational therapist who is the Program Director of an adult psychiatric partial hospital. On September 11, 2001, she was vacationing in Strasbourg, France. As a result, she made frequent trips to Ground Zero upon her return to New York, to validate that what seemed unbelievable had occured. Photography and graphic arts are avocational pursuits, and her work has been published in books about French waterways as well as in this volume.

Donna Brennan is a lifelong resident of Fort Lee, NJ. She is a freelance photojournalist for several New Jersey publications and newspapers. Donna also serves as a member of both the Fort Lee Film Commission and the Fort Lee Historic Committee. Donna's work on the film commission includes research and restoration of silent films made in Fort Lee during Fort Lee's days as the motion picture capital of the world. Donna also works with digital technology and production for public access programming, film festivals and retrospectives and the production of newsletters. She is proud to be associated with this book.

Ann Burkhardt, MA, OTR/L, FAOTA, BCN, is the Director of Occupational Therapy at NYPH-Columbia Presbyterian Hospital in New York City. She is on the faculty of both Columbia University and Mercy College (Dobbs Ferry). Ann is currently serving as Director of the American Occupational Therapy Association. She is a Past-President of the New York State Occupational Therapy Association. As a clinician, Ann has a wellness-focused community-based private practice with cancer survivors in Manhattan and Long Island, NY. She is a published author of several books and peer-reviewed journal articles on topics ranging from oncology rehabilitation and stroke rehabilitation to complementary care and alternative medicine. An administrator, leader, educator, community activist and advocate, Ann has lived and worked in New York City for over 20 years.

Hanna Diamond, MA, OTR, has been a practicing therapist for over 20 years. She has worked primarily with the psychosocial needs of those individuals with psychiatric illnesses, and has recently addressed the needs pertaining to the homeless and disabled and survivors of domestic violence.

Mary V. Donohue, PhD, OT, FAOTA, is Clinical Professor at the Department of Occupational Therapy at New York University. She teaches courses in psychiatric conditions, psychosocial assessment and intervention, and a community fieldwork seminar. She is the co-chair of the MNYD Research Committee, and has developed the *Group Profile* to assess levels of group function.

Brad Gottlieb is a senior at Hewlett High School and has always had a very strong connection with animals. Brad remembers working for his father, a veterinarian, ever since he was a boy and enjoyed attending his father's Veterinary Medicine courses at Farmingdale University. He has been a volunteer Junior Firefighter at the Hewlett Fire House since 1997 and when called to Ground Zero, helped with the K-9 Unit.

Naomi Greenberg, OTR, MPH, PhD, FAOTA, is Director of the Occupational Therapy Assistant Program at LaGuardia Community College. Her biography is included in *Who's Who in Medicine and Health Care 2002-2003*. She has traveled extensively to almost 80 countries on five continents where she was able to directly observe diversity in spirituality. Her interests are broad, ranging from having held an experimental course combining offenders and college students at a prison to teaching refugees during a sabbatical year fellowship leave in Italy. She remains a true believer in the therapeutic value of occupation.

Iris Kimberg, MS, PT, OTR, is a long-time resident of Lower Manhattan, and has owned many successful therapy businesses downtown since 1979. She is currently doing consulting and lecturing in the field to both physical therapy and occupational therapy students and therapists.

Sabina Luna is a senior in the Occupational Therapy Program at York College of the City University of New York. She is an immigrant from Bangladesh and has been in the United States for eleven years. She is the youngest of nine siblings. Her father was a renowned lawyer. She is very happily married with two wonderful children.

Frank Pascarelli is a former firefighter, and Occupational Therapist with Children's Healthcare of Atlanta, and Advanced Rehab Services as well as a consultant on workplace and school violence prevention/intervention. He is also in the Air Force Reserves, serving as a Biomedical Science Corps Officer with the 96th Surgical Operations Squadron at Eglin Air Force Base. He served during the Gulf War as part of a Combat Stress Control team. Pascarelli was sent to New York to conduct a needs assessment and to provide crisis intervention in the post 9/11 period.

Jennifer Persh, MA, received her degree in occupational therapy from New York University. She was the recipient of the 2002 President's Service Award for Volunteerism and Community Service for her work with Project Liberty. Jennifer graduated from the University of Michigan with a Bachelor of Arts in Psychology, where she was a member of Psi Chi, the National Honor Society in Psychology. Jennifer is currently employed as an occupational therapist at St. Mary's Hospital for Children in Bayside, New York and resides in Manhattan.

Jane Prawda, MA, OTR, MS/Ed, received her MA in 1987 from New York University in Occupational Therapy. She received her MS in 1981 from C.W. Post in Special Education/Elementary Education Certification. She received her BA in 1979 from Hofstra University in Psychology. She is a member of Psi Chi and Phi Beta Kappa. She was the Metropolitan New York District Membership Chair from 1992-1993. She worked as a Senior Occupational Therapist from 1989-1995 within the Department of Psychiatry in Pain Management and Post Traumatic Stress Disorder at the Lenox Hill Hospital in New York. She contributed to *Freedom from Chronic Pain,* co-authored with Norman J. Marcus, MD, and Jean S. Arbeiter. She currently works as a Pediatric Occupational Therapist.

Helen Rosenstark was born in Poland where she survived the Holocaust as one of the hidden children. Her remarks: "I was just standing next to the author, Naomi Greenberg, and took the pictures."

Anne Hiller Scott, PhD, OTR, FAOTA, is Assistant Professor, Founder and Director of the Division of Occupational Therapy at Long Island University, Brooklyn Campus. She is a frequent presenter at international, national and state venues, most recently presenting on topics related to health promotion and culture, community practice and issues of concern for consumers with mental health and physical disability problems. With over three decades of experience, she has written numerous chapters and articles on occupational therapy on mental health, community health, and wellness. She edited the book *New Frontiers in Psychosocial Occupational Therapy.* She is a Fellow of the American Occupational Therapy Association, a member of the national education honor society, Kappa Delta Pi, and serves on six professional and community organization boards.

Mary Squillace BA, BS/MS, OTR/L, has been a practicing Occupational Therapist for seven years. Mary's teaching experiences include the creation and presentation of the seminar "Reality 101" to graduating students, focusing on the transition from student life to practicing professionals; being Assistant Professor at Long Island University for a practical anatomy lab; presenting and organizing seminars in Advanced Clinical Neurology for Touro College, the Manhattan Campus; teaching seminars in anatomy, kinesiology, physiology, emergency procedures, musculoskeletal injuries, and exercise programming for healthy people; and special populations seminars for the East Coast Instructor Training School associated with the World Fitness Alliance at various national sites. Clinically, Mary has worked at several medical centers located within the New York City and Long Island regions with a focus on traumatic brain injury, spinal cord injury and acute care. Mary is currently working within an outpatient care facility with a focus on hand therapy and home-based early intervention. Mary has volunteered at youth centers in New York City assisting in activities for children and teens who are limited due to physical and psychosocial disabilities; for the Nassau County Special Olympics Committee preparing and training young adults, teens and children with a variety of disabilities in athletics and competitive games; and for Hofstra University Athletic Advantage organizing and preparing athletic training demonstrations for adult athletes focusing on the variety of training techniques for safe and effective workouts and successful competitions.

Diane B. Tewfik, MA, OTR/L, is Associate Professor and fieldwork coordinator at York College of the City University of New York. She is a founding member and co-chair since 1995 of the Metropolitan New York District of the New York State Occupational Therapy Association's Mental Health Task Force. This task force, as part of the Mental Health Special Interest Group, has been acclaimed locally as well as nationally for its work in consumer advocacy, promotion of cost-effective models, networking, and marketing of the profession. In 1997, she was awarded the New York State Occupational Therapy Association's Merit of Practice Award in the area of mental health practice. She has published widely and presented at numerous conferences locally, nationally, and internationally.

Jennifer Wright, MS, OTR, NZROT, is an occupational therapist with 20 years of experience working in the United States. She taught most recently at the University of Indianapolis School of Occupational Therapy. Having spent a good deal of her life as a single parent, working and raising two fantastic children, she decided in 1999 to find adventure for herself. Always an outdoor lover, she chose to go to New Zealand where she teaches at Otago Polytechnic School of Occupational Therapy. She has met her soul mate and has created a simpler life with spinning, organic gardening, and a great deal of laughter. She also has a personal and coaching business, The Wright Direction.

Foreword

It was a call that I had been almost expecting, and when it came I was relieved. Like many bystanders of the tragic events of 9/11, I had felt the need to contribute to the recovery effort. As an occupational therapy educator, my skills are writing and speaking and it was that call that set in motion the groundwork for presenting the stories that appear in this volume.

Debbie Berenson, the Public Relations chairperson for the local Occupational Therapy (OT) association, was calling on behalf of the planning committee for OT Week. It is a longstanding tradition that the Metropolitan New York District (MNYD) Occupational Therapy Association of the New York State Occupational Therapy Association (NYSOTA) contact the New York City Mayor's office in anticipation of OT week. The Mayor's Office issues a proclamation officially declaring Occupational Therapy Week. The official proclamation is presented by a representative of the Mayor's office at a membership meeting held each April. At that time there is also a presentation featuring a topic of vital professional interest for the members.

Debbie and her co-chair on the Public Relations Committee, Charles Grey, thought that I would be able to rise to the challenge of a presentation on the psychological aspects of 9/11. I was approached because of my involvement in many educational activities in psychosocial occupational therapy, in community health, and wellness. When Debbie called, we spoke briefly of the emotional impact of serious physical disabilities and how psychological wounds often last longer than physical wounds. Many therapists do not see the full picture of psychological recovery nor do health care resources necessarily fund this aspect of healing.

[Haworth co-indexing entry note]: "Foreword." Scott, Anne Hiller. Co-published simultaneously in *Occupational Therapy in Mental Health* (The Haworth Press, Inc.) Vol. 19, No. 3/4, 2003, pp. xxiii-xxx; and: *Surviving 9/11: Impact and Experiences of Occupational Therapy Practitioners* (ed: Pat Precin) The Haworth Press, Inc., 2003, pp. xix-xxvi. Single or multiple copies of this article are available for a fee from The Haworth Document Delivery Service [1-800-HAWORTH, 9:00 a.m. - 5:00 p.m. (EST). E-mail address: docdelivery@haworthpress. com].

Mental health parity, and equal coverage for psychological stress, has emerged as a major concern in the context of the aftermath of 9/11.

The outcome of our conversation was a panel presentation held in NYC on April 10, 2002 at Mt. Sinai Hospital. The Mayor's Proclamation was read by Debbie Berenson (see Appendix 1) and I introduced the evening's focus followed by each of the six presenters.

THE THEME–POST 9/11: PERSONAL AND PROFESSIONAL PERSPECTIVES

When I was asked to address 9/11, I felt that it would be difficult to do justice to this topic without looking at both the personal impact of this event as well as the professional involvement. Hence the title, "Post 9/11: Personal and Professional Perspectives." It seemed imperative to acknowledge the personal toll this event generated. We are people first and professionals second. So many of us were profoundly overwhelmed by this horrific attack, which immersed our city, our nation's capital, and indeed the world in its staggering personal, social, economic, spiritual, and political aftershocks. To this day and for generations to come the losses will be both personal and professional for the people of our city who come from all walks of life and diverse backgrounds reflecting our international community, and our grief has become the nation's grief.

To present a broad overview on the panel, I wanted to include as many practice areas as possible, since no one escaped the impact of this devastating attack. I believed that a panel presentation would be the best venue to bring together interested therapists. I immediately contacted several people who gladly offered to participate and to represent some of the many dimensions of 9/11. Iris Kimberg, MS, OTR, PT, discussed the needs of therapists (occupational, physical and speech therapists) in the Downtown area whose practices were damaged in the aftermath (Johansson, 2001). A therapist from New York/Cornell Hospital, Robin Silver, provided the perspective of the major burn unit in New York City (NYC). A dance therapist, Christine Zimbelmann, and occupational therapist, Joanne Cordero of St. Vincent's Hospital and Medical Center, spoke to community mental health issues in the short term, and dealing with ongoing outreach to firefighters in the community. Cheryl King of St. Luke's-Roosevelt received a grant from the United Hospital Fund to address the needs of those with serious mental illness to prevent further isolation and social withdrawal. Pat Precin, affiliated with the

Brooklyn Bureau of Community Service, spoke of a program this agency developed to assist displaced workers.

WINTER, THEN SPRING

To introduce the evening I used the theme taken from the title of a local memorial (Coming Together to Heal, 2002), "Winter, Then Spring." I described the beauty of a spring day the previous April weekend. The street I live on was enveloped in a canopy of puffy white pear blossoms, the air was perfumed with the tropical scent of hyacinth, and the entrance to the Promenade revealed scores of lavender azalea and golden daffodils in regal splendor–*Spring*. The Promenade in Brooklyn Heights looks over the East River and the Manhattan skyline. I always shudder now at the skyline, looking for the ghost of a proud edifice no longer present, the Twin Towers–*Winter*.

Our destination was to view a newly planted garden at the foot of the Brooklyn shore. The planting was in the shape of two long rectangles, representing the World Trade Center Twin Towers. In the garden were several children and adults, and two firefighters. To the side was a fire engine from the local firehouse, Engine 205 and Ladder 118, which had lost eight men in the blast. As I watched this group tend the garden–I thought that they had found their occupational therapy–a small way to find meaning through this special occupation of gardening and to pay tribute to those lost in a brutal and senseless act that left indescribable desolation in its wake.

There were 25,000 daffodils in that garden–part of the Daffodil Project (*www.partnerships*). This project was part of an international outpouring of goodwill. A Dutch grower, Hans van Waardenburg of B&K Bulbs, and the city of Rotterdam, and the Netherlands Chamber of Commerce donated 1.8 million bulbs to NYC (*www.parkscouncil*). This particular memorial was designed by the Brooklyn Bridge Park Coalition, and the sign in front read "Winter, Then Spring," their title for this act of healing and recovery.

As I continued my introduction, I gave a brief overview of the news of the previous weeks (almost six months to the day post- 9/11). The bombing of the World Trade Center (WTC) had struck every chord of life in the city. The news reported on unemployment, environmental pollution, counseling for firefighters (the numbers seeking help had tripled over the previous year's statistics), transportation disruptions, and the slow economic recovery. I did not touch on the ultimate personal loss of life and the struggle of loved ones to come to terms with these untimely deaths. For those living or working in New York City, every aspect of daily life has been disrupted for our beloved community–we truly had come to appreciate the role of habits and loss of normalcy in our daily routines.

Winter came early in September of 2001, it struck suddenly on the morning of 9/11. It was swift, unexpected, and very bitter–leaving desolation, despair, and destruction in a matter of moments. For some survivors the shroud of winter remains–there is no spring–yet. Part of our commitment as therapists and citizens must be to help generate the resilience and coping needed to move on. As a therapist committed to community health, I closed my comments raising concerns around the need to address mental health parity. Long after physical rehabilitation is complete, psychic scars remain. Post-traumatic stress can be an enduring crippling disorder, as has been noted in the literature related to the bombing in Oklahoma City. Coverage for depression or complicated bereavement is only the beginning of a healing process, and one should not equate the healing of the human spirit with the ticking of a meter measuring hours and minutes of therapy available. We all have a role to play in advocating for these basic human needs.

POSTSCRIPT:
A PERSONAL PERSPECTIVE OF A 9/11 SURVIVOR

Another professional presentation–the same local OT Association, MNYD of NYSOTA that sponsored the 9/11 program, hosted the NYSOTA Conference on a fall weekend of 2002 at Long Island University (LIU). The theme for the conference was "Restoration and Renewal."

The keynote speaker was a WTC survivor, Lauren Manning, who sustained burns over 80% of her body. The story of her recovery has been chronicled by her husband Greg Manning (2002). Her personal courage and determination were inspiring. Her recovery was nurtured in large part by the skill and dedication of occupational therapists at the burn center of New York Hospital Cornell Medical Center and through the expertise and sensitivity of the occupational therapists at Burke Rehabilitation Center. Ms. Manning's unique perspective spoke to the importance of hope and trust conveyed by her occupational therapists–who from the beginning helped her past innumerable painful hurdles in a journey to recovery which is measured in seconds of pain leading to gains that will be measured over several years. One year post-injury, she is just starting a series of several hand surgeries to regain some use of her right hand, and her home care therapy is provided on a daily basis.

The quality of her care addressed both the compelling emotional and physical needs secondary to her injury and its circumstances. The engagement of Ms. Manning was focused through the goals that she valued, and her motivation stemmed from the desire to move on with her life–to be there for her son and husband and for her colleagues (close to 70% of the staff at Cantor-Fitzgerald perished). Left with one word to describe her–I would say determination. She continues to engage in a valiant battle moment to moment to regain her life. Her faith in what she has gained through occupational therapy is so strong that she acknowledges the importance of sharing her experience with the public as a dedicated advocate.

As I was leaving Ms. Manning's presentation, I encountered a member of the staff at LIU who had been severely burned over 75% of his body in the Trade Towers. He had seen Ms. Manning enter the building and knew who she was and why she had come. He had never discussed his personal condition with me. He disclosed that he, too, had a very long and painful recovery. Unlike Ms. Manning, there were times of deep despair when suicide felt like the best option. With support from family, he weathered these dark and life-threatening storms. His ultimate inspiration was another person with a devastating disability who was moving on with his life.

I was struck by the differences of these two survivors. No two people are alike–but there are common needs and common causes that we must recognize. On a daily basis, therapists encounter individuals dealing with the catastrophic impact of a serious illness–be it physical and/or emotional. For individual clients, their lifestyle and spirit may be shattered–daily routines and interactions with family, work, and social ties may be completely disrupted–and in some cases never resumed. We in New York have had a small dose of this in our experience with the aftermath of 9/11. Unfortunately, however, therapists do not always have the view of the full spectrum of the disability experience–being privy only to a brief temporal glimpse–an acute or subacute hospitalization, or a few sessions of home care. "Our contacts may be extensive, but often they are brief and only partially fulfilled" (Fine, 1991, p. 493), a tragic example of the failure of not meeting long-term outcomes for individuals with serious physical disabilities–75% do not work, and the figure for those with mental illness is closer to 85%.

It makes one wonder where the rehabilitation is–if our most involved clients are the least likely to return to the mainstream of life. "Evidence suggests that we may already have reframed the rehabilitation process to fit today's economy rather than to fit today's patients" (Fine, 1991, p. 501). New Yorkers have sustained themselves in a major catastrophe and continue to work towards achieving normalcy. Mayor Giuliani made headlines for encouraging us to resume our daily routines–work, play, leisure, travel, spirituality, family, and social life. These common place occupations have curative potential–as any occupational therapist knows. But perhaps there is a compelling need to educate others about our value to society. The disaster of 9/11 gave us a unique view of a catastrophic tragedy to a major and once thriving metropolis and how its vitality is recovering through engagement, one meaningful activity at a time.

In the aftermath of 9/11 it is obvious that the mental health needs are staggering (Chiles, 2002). In the metropolitan New York area, a survey of families who lost loved ones indicates that they have experienced a 40% drop in their income and over three quarters may need mental health counseling (Storm, 2002). It was predicted that job-related needs will be handled by the end of 2003. However, mental health needs will require $44 million in 2004, and these needs will be ongoing.

A New York City Board of Education survey found 15% (107,000 children) have agoraphobia related to 9/11. There are 1 million children in the New York City school system and in this survey of a sample of 8,000, 87% demonstrated at least one symptom of post-traumatic stress disorder (Campanile, 2002). The study concluded that about 200,000 students in the school system have serious mental health problems. Other emotional concerns documented were increased incidence of separation anxiety, panic disorders, conduct disorders, generalized anxiety, major depression and a rate of post-traumatic stress disorder that is over five times the rate for the American student population. A study of adults, published in April, reported that one in three New Yorkers displayed symptoms of post-traumatic stress (Geller, 4/7/02).

Another New Yorker, Susan B. Fine, who delivered the Eleanor Clarke Slagle lecture in 1991, studied survivors. This lecture reviewed "Resilience and Human Adaptability: Who Rises Above Adversity?" Fine cautions therapists against taking the "snapshot approach" (p. 500) to working with individuals whose needs are multifaceted. If ever the need presented itself to apply the truism of working with the "whole person," this is the opportunity. It is also true that many of the physical and psychological wounds secondary to 9/11 will require years to resolve. It is therefore important to put forth a steadfast advocacy for programs that continue to help survivors of 9/11 for as long as help is needed. Part of the proceeds of this book has been devoted to such.

The program was one of those transcendent moments when tales of grief, fear, courage, hope, determination, professional devotion, and leadership inspired a sense of awe. The response to the panel was overwhelming. It was decided immediately to share our perspectives with a broader audience. Mary Donohue, co-editor of *Occupational Therapy in Mental Health* (*OTMH*), acknowledged the significance of this presentation and suggested that this could become a book. One of the panelists, Pat Precin, eagerly came forward to volunteer as editor and the text began to take form.

Anne Hiller Scott

REFERENCES

Campanile, C. (2002, May 2). The silent victims–kids–9 out of 10 traumatized months later. *New York Post,* p. 8.

Chiles, N. (2002, May 2). Enduring pain study: City students feeling trauma months after Sept. 11. *Newsday,* p. A3. *Coming together to heal.* (n.d.). Retrieved April 10, 2002, from *http://www.thirteen.org/nyvoices/highlights/garden.html*

The Daffodil Project 2001. Making New York City bloom again. (n.d.). Retrieved April 10, 2002, from *http://www.parkscouncil.org/daffodils.html*

The Daffodil Project, Fall 2001. Volunteers make New York City bloom again. (n.d.) Retrieved April 10, 2002, from *http://www.partnerships for parks.org/youdo/youdo/_daffodils.html*

Fine, S. B. (1991). Resilience and human adaptability: Who rises above adversity? *American Journal of Occupational Therapy, 45* (6), 493-503.

Geller, A. (2002, April 7). Post-9/11 stress rising. *New York Post,* p. 22.

Johansson, C. (2001, November 20). *New York OTs and PTs need your help.* Retrieved April 8, 2001, from *http://www.aota.org/nonmembers/area1/links/link219.asp*

Manning, G. (2002). *Love, Greg and Lauren. A powerful, true story of courage, hope, and survival.* New York: Bantam Books.

Storm, S. (2002, July 8). 9/11 victims need $768 million in aid into 2003, study says. *New York Times,* p. B3.

APPENDIX 1.
The Mayor's Proclamation written by Debbie Berenson
and now in public domain.

Office of the Mayor
City of New York

Proclamation

Whereas: Occupational Therapy week is being observed by the Metropolitan New York District of the Occupational Therapy Association from the eighth through the twelfth of April; and

Whereas: The year's theme for the observance is "Post 9/11: Personal and Professional Perspectives," honoring Occupational Therapists and Occupational Therapy Assistants who have made vital contributions to the rehabilitation of survivors of the terrorist attack on the World Trade Center, and people who were affected by the attack. Many of these educated professionals have worked with injured people, burn victims, firefighters, police officers, members of other uniformed services, medical personnel, and rescuers; as well as with those otherwise affected by the tragic events on and following September 11th. Occupational Therapy professionals provide injured patients with individualized exercise programs that help them achieve maximum functional mobility, and teach techniques that enable patients to function as independently as possible at home and in the community. For patients suffering from trauma, therapists offer psychosocial support groups, coping strategies, therapeutic listening, and relaxation exercises that help them deal with their individual circumstances and continue to lead productive lives. In addition, members of the Metropolitan New York District are assisting colleagues whose practices in lower Manhattan were affected by the tragedy; and

Whereas: working in public and private health care facilities, schools, rehabilitation centers, community agencies, hospitals, nursing homes, and in the community, Occupational Therapists and Occupational Therapy Assistants are vital members of the healthcare team, working with doctors, nurses, and physical therapists, social workers, and others to maximize each patient's recovery. Each year many New Yorkers of all ages benefit from their skills and compassion.

Now therefore, I Michael R. Bloomberg, Mayor of The City of New York, in recognition of this important annual observance, do hereby proclaim the week of April 8-12, 2002 in the city of New York as

"Occupational Therapy Week"

Michael R. Bloomberg
Mayor
In witness whereof I have hereunto
Set my hand and caused the seal of
The City of New York to be affixed.

Introduction:
Surviving 9/11:
Impact and Experiences
of Occupational Therapy Practitioners

Pat Precin, MS, OTR/L

American Airlines Flight 77 departed from Dallas International Airport carrying 64 passengers en route to Los Angeles. At approximately 9:46 a.m., September 11, 2001, the hijacked plane crashed into the West Side of the Pentagon building creating a gaping wound 65 yards wide. One hundred and twenty-five people died and 80 were injured. Evidence indicated that the terrorists' true destination might have been the White House.

On September 11, 2001, forty passengers rebelled against four al Qaeda terrorists in a three-foot wide aisle aboard a Boeing 757 traveling from Newark to San Francisco at 35,000 feet. The plane, United Airlines Flight 93, crashed into a reclaimed strip-mining field in Shanksville, Pennsylvania near the Stonycreek K-12 School where 500 students and staff were beginning a new school year. Two hundred and twenty-four people were murdered at both sites.

Over 2,800 more people were murdered when, on September 11, 2001, terrorists hijacked two planes and crashed them into the World Trade Center Towers. At 8:46 a.m., American Airlines Flight 11 hit the

[Haworth co-indexing entry note]: "Introduction: Surviving 9/11: Impact and Experiences of Occupational Therapy Practitioners." Precin, Pat. Co-published simultaneously in *Occupational Therapy in Mental Health* (The Haworth Press, Inc.) Vol. 19, No. 3/4, 2003, pp. 1-4 and: *Surviving 9/11: Impact and Experiences of Occupational Therapy Practitioners* (ed: Pat Precin) The Haworth Press, Inc., 2003, pp. 1-4. Single or multiple copies of this article are available for a fee from The Haworth Document Delivery Service [1-800-HAWORTH, 9:00 a.m. - 5:00 p.m. (EST). E-mail address: docdelivery@haworthpress.com].

http://www.haworthpress.com/web/OTMH
Digital Object Identifier: 10.1300/J004v19n03_01

North Tower and at 9:03 a.m., United Airlines Flight 175 hit the South Tower. By 9:59 a.m., the South Tower had collapsed and by 10:29 a.m., the North Tower fell to the ground. A total of seven buildings were destroyed in New York City and many additional structures were damaged, resulting in a 20-acre void referred to as Ground Zero. More than 1.8 million tons of debris were removed, but nothing compared to the loss of lives.

How could occupational therapy practitioners (OTPs) help themselves and the people of New York, Pennsylvania, Washington, DC, and the country as a whole resume functioning? They stayed after hours to provide aggressive manual therapy, splints, wound care and scar management in order to prevent adhesions in burn survivors so they might have a chance to walk and use their hands again. They helped a Senior Vice President who escaped from the 103rd floor of Tower Two resume work from her ergonomically modified home and begin teaching restorative yoga classes. They analyzed the job market and found work for people who lost their livelihoods. They worked with FEMA's Project Liberty to provide disaster mental health counseling to people in homeless shelters and psychiatric clinics. They taught people with disabilities how to set up individualized emergency plans. They wrote grants to create and implement otherwise non-fundable programs. They created community-quilting projects. They worked with firefighters from Ground Zero who had difficulty expressing their feelings. They gave guidance and support to their occupational therapy students so they could continue their studies. They performed a Ground Zero needs assessment. They incorporated much-needed psychosocial interventions with their physically disabled clients. They learned much about post-traumatic stress disorder, acute trauma reaction, and normal responses to trauma. They established a relief fund for occupational and physical therapists whose businesses had been impacted by the attacks. They performed home visits with Muslim families and worked with children. They expressed their feelings while creating flag pins that raised money for the survivors of 9/11. They spoke of and developed spiritual spontaneity.

This book chronicles the events and experiences of OTPs dealing with the 9/11 disaster and its aftermath. Their personal and professional narratives describe what it was like the day of the tragedy (Part I: September 11th: Day One), the Ground Zero Milieu (Part II), and the role of Spirituality (Part III) in their own healing process and in the process of healing others. Intimate accounts accented by interspersed photographs unfold the horror, humanity, fear, reverence, turmoil, spirit, drive, and compassion of the time.

The healing aspect of storytelling is very powerful. People told of their experiences and/or thoughts about the attacks over and over again. It is now a year later and people are still sharing stories with each other. Editing this book was very therapeutic. It presented the opportunity to focus on what happened, to organize an otherwise disorganized frightening traumatic event, and to experience the personal growth and healing of many of the chapter contributors as they wrote and reworked their material. While a national call for chapters was posted, many OTPs were approached to write because of their known direct involvement with 9/11, but many declined because they were still too emotionally raw. Some offered photographs instead.

This is the first of two volumes edited by Pat Precin about 9/11 and the impact and experiences of OTPs. The second, also published by The Haworth Press, Inc., discusses various programs and interventions created and implemented by OTPs to help survivors of 9/11. It also explores the role of creativity in the healing process of practitioners and their clients.

ACKNOWLEDGMENTS

I would like to acknowledge all of the authors for their contributions, not only for their written chapters but also for their invaluable, creative, selfless work with people in need after the tragedy of September 11th. I am grateful to the victims/survivors/heroes of 9/11 for granting permission to publish their experiences and for sharing their stories. Anne Hiller Scott, after being requested by Debbie Berenson, coordinated the panel presentation for the Mayor's Proclamation Ceremony that inspired this book, and she wrote the foreword. The following people helped concretize images of 9/11 through their photographic contributions or artwork: Fran Babiss, PhD, OTR/L; Donna Brennan, of Fort Lee, New Jersey; Gilad Rosner; Helen Rosenstark; Naomi Greenberg, OTR, MPH, PhD, FAOTA; and Mary Donohue, PhD, OT, FAOTA. It was a pleasure working with Mary Donohue and Marie-Louise Blount in the preparation of this manuscript. Marilyn Maxwell, PhD, English instructor at Hewlett High School, provided her student Brad Gottlieb's college entrance essay on 9/11 and provided encouragement throughout the completion of this book. Peter LaBarbera provided ongoing support. Part of the proceeds of this publication will be donated to two programs that continue to help people affected by 9/11: "Reach Out and Have Some Fun," a program for psychiatric clients at St. Luke's/Roosevelt Hospital in New York City conducted by Occupational and Creative Arts Therapists and detailed in this book, and "Weaving the Community Together," a quilting project conducted by the Occupational Therapy Assistant Program of the State University of New York's Orange County Community College.

SEPTEMBER 11th DAY ONE:
PHOTOS

PHOTO 1. Both Towers Are Hit.

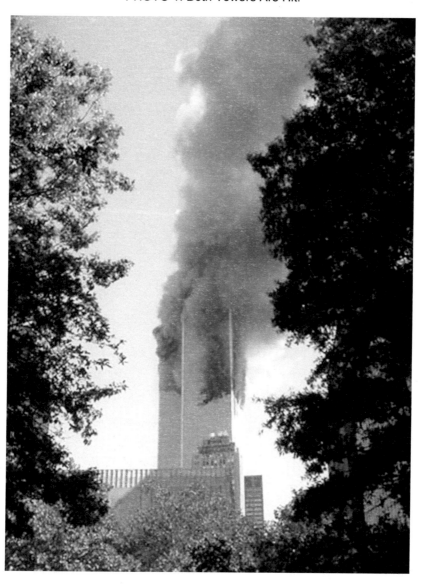

Photo by Gilad Rosner. Used by permission.

PHOTO 2. The Twin Towers Continue to Burn.

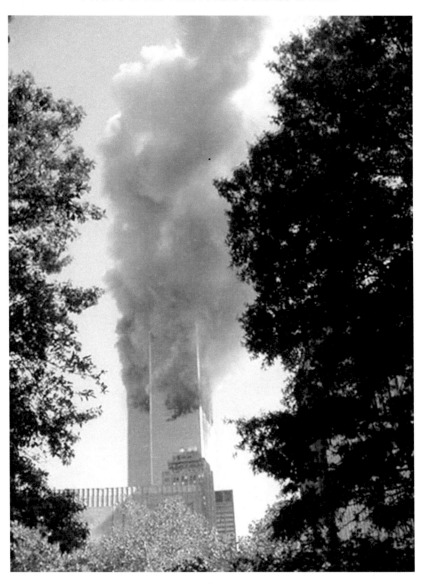

Photo by Gilad Rosner. Used by permission.

PHOTO 3.

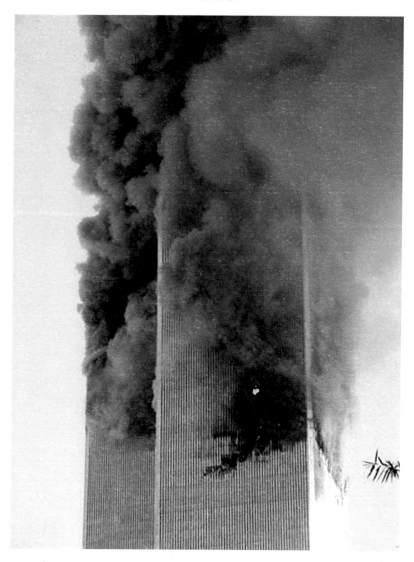

PHOTO 4.

Photo by Gilad Rosner. Used by permission.

PHOTO 5.

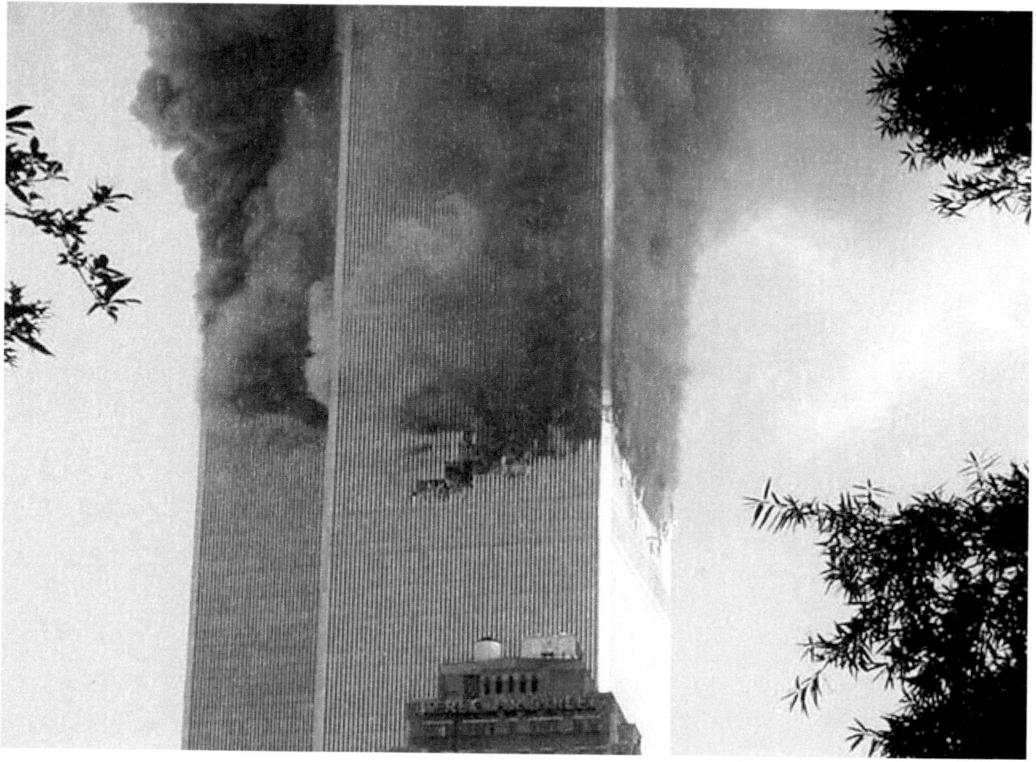

Photo by Gilad Rosner. Used by permission.

PHOTO 6.

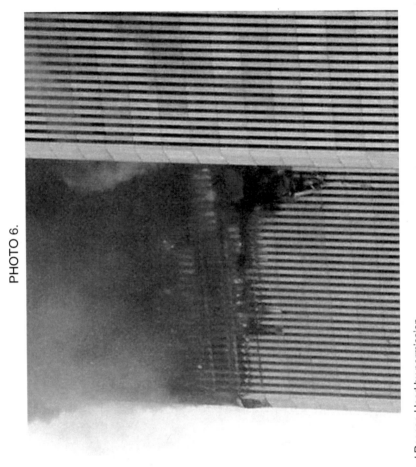

PHOTO 7.

Photo by Gilad Rosner. Used by permission.

PHOTO 8. People Running from Manhattan into Brooklyn over the Brooklyn Bridge.

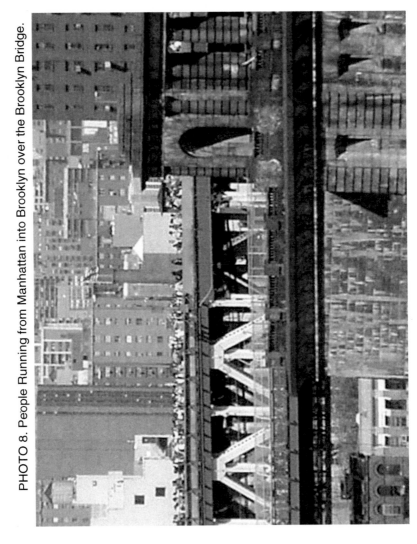

PHOTO 9. People Continuing to Escape.

Photo by Gilad Rosner. Used by permission.

PHOTO 10. Almost Everyone Has Crossed Over the Bridge.

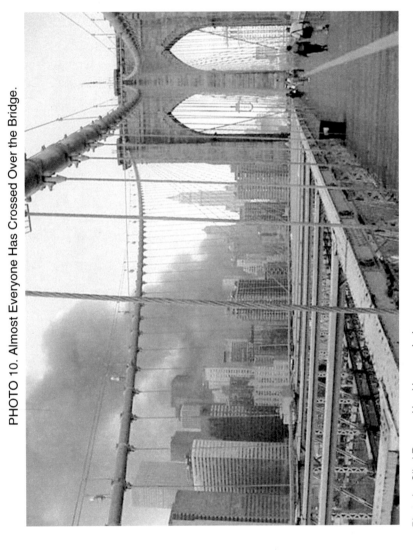

PHOTO 11. Smoke Darkens and Thickens.

Photo by Gilad Rosner. Used by permission.

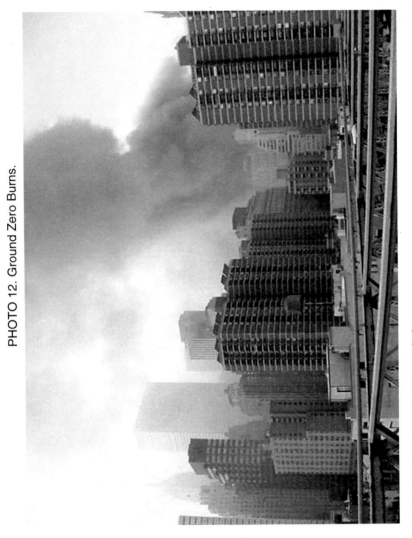

PHOTO 12. Ground Zero Burns.

Photo by Gilad Rosner. Used by permission.

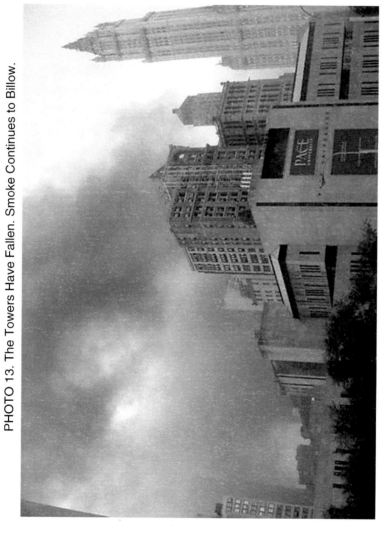

PHOTO 13. The Towers Have Fallen. Smoke Continues to Billow.

Photo by Gilad Rosner. Used by permission.

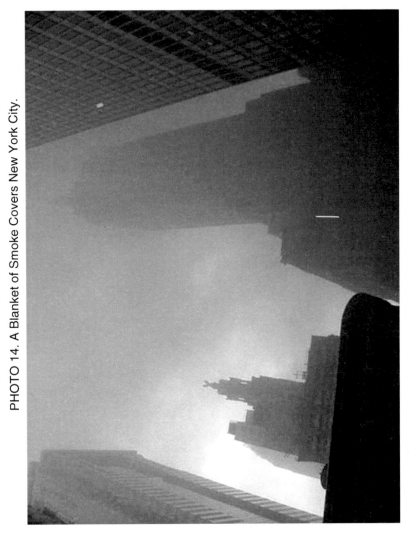

PHOTO 14. A Blanket of Smoke Covers New York City.

Photo by Gilad Rosner. Used by permission.

PHOTO 15. Obscured Sun

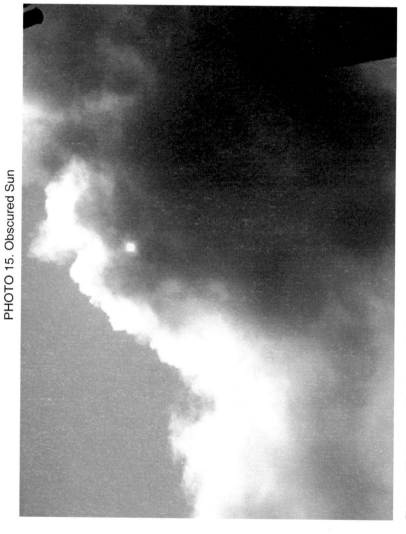

PHOTO 16. A Dark City

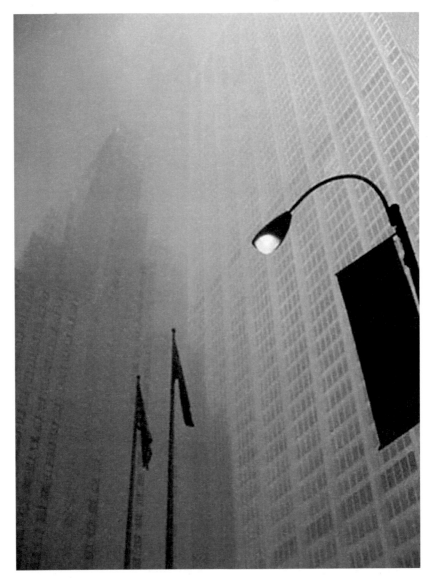

Photo by Gilad Rosner. Used by permission.

"When it gets dark enough you can see the stars."–Lee Salk

PART I:
SEPTEMBER 11th: DAY ONE

From the 103rd Floor

Mary Squillace, BA, BS/MS, OTR/L

It couldn't be. I heard a boom and felt my building shake. As I looked outside my window on the 103rd floor of 2 World Trade Center on September 11, a massive fireball seemed to rise from the ground. The sight filled me with horror. Even in my office, I could feel the heat on my cheeks. (Wein & Rhodes, 2001, p. 82)

Judy Wein, senior vice president for a financial consulting company, was in her office on the 103rd floor of 2 World Trade Center on the morning of September 11th. This is her story of survival and her experience with Occupational Therapy services.

[Haworth co-indexing entry note]: "From the 103rd Floor." Squillace, Mary. Co-published simultaneously in *Occupational Therapy in Mental Health* (The Haworth Press, Inc.) Vol. 19, No. 3/4, 2003, pp. 23-26; and: *Surviving 9/11: Impact and Experiences of Occupational Therapy Practitioners* (ed: Pat Precin) The Haworth Press, Inc., 2003, pp. 23-26. Single or multiple copies of this article are available for a fee from The Haworth Document Delivery Service [1-800-HAWORTH, 9:00 a.m. - 5:00 p.m. (EST). E-mail address: docdelivery@haworthpress.com].

http://www.haworthpress.com/web/OTMH
Digital Object Identifier: 10.1300/J004v19n03_02

23

On September 11th, Judy was at her desk at approximately 7:15 a.m. At the time of the impact of the first plane into Tower One, she said she felt her building shake. She immediately jumped out of her seat and shouted, "Get out of here!" She and some of her co-workers walked from the 103rd floor to the 78th floor, where they decided to attempt to take an elevator down. At this time, a message over the public announcement system broadcasted they were secure. While others felt that it was safe to return to their desks, she thought she heard that it was safe to leave via the elevators. On the 78th floor, while waiting for the elevator amongst a larger than usual crowd, there was an enormous explosion. Judy was thrown across the floor. At this time, she thought, *Oh my God. Is this the end? Are we going to make it?* Judy stated, "My mind was preparing itself to remain calm." When the confusion decreased, she called out to her boss, but the only response she heard was a co-worker who called out to her, "We are over here." As she followed the voices of the surviving, ambulatory people, she recalls stepping over many bodies. Then she saw her boss, unconscious and crushed by a huge piece of marble. Judy had worked with him for over 20 years and considered him one of her best friends. She also saw another co-worker with his lower extremities crushed under a large slab of marble. When she approached her boss, she saw that he was conscious. Judy tried to remove the marble piece with her uninjured arm, but he cried out in pain and told her to leave it there. She stated that he said a final "I love you" to the group of co-workers waiting for the elevator. There was nothing that she could do but hope that the emergency medical system workers would come soon to help him. Judy stated that she began to feel confused about what was happening around her. She stated, "I was basically sitting there, bewildered, and not knowing what to do. I knew that I should do something, but just did not know what to do. I felt, not an urgency, but a pulling to get out of there."

She was now rejoined by three of her co-workers and they decided that they would continue to walk down as far as they could. At the time of the impact into the second tower, Judy suffered a shattered ulna, three broken ribs, a punctured lung, and a trauma to her head. Needless to say she was bleeding, but without pain while walking down the flights. She recalled that as they were walking down, there were firefighters and rescue workers walking up. At the 40th floor, a security guard told her to rest. "I could not sit down. I had to continue. Something was telling me to keep moving. When I tried to sit, it was like something was pushing me back up," Judy stated. They reached the 40th floor and were told by the rescue workers to take the elevator down to the lower level. Once that elevator reached the basement of the towers and the passengers walked off, the doors closed and the elevator continued up to its next destination. That was the last trip of that elevator. As they finally reached the outside, she was put into an ambulance and as the ambulance was pulling away, Judy watched out the back window as her tower went down. At that time, she thought, *Oh my God, this is the end of my co-workers.* Judy recalls remaining calm throughout the entire episode, but then, as she watched the building collapse, she felt very sad and had a sense of vast loss and emotional pain.

Judy was taken to a New York hospital where they performed exploratory surgery for her internal bleeding, surgery on her arm and stitched her head wound. She recalls her encounters with each of her Occupational Therapists, from her bedside Occupational Therapist to her outpatient Occupational Therapists.

Judy reported having post-traumatic stress disorder following this event. She admitted to having panic attacks when sitting in traffic on a bridge, overhearing stories about the tragedy, and at the thought of traveling by air. There was a time when the fire alarm was set off while she was in therapy, and she recalled having an overwhelming flashback of being on the 78th floor at the time of impact. She said that she thought that she might be thrown across the room. So she left therapy, walked 13 blocks until she found the subway, and then felt safe. She had difficulty watching the news or reading the newspaper for some time thereafter. "There was all of this awful news coming out at me, so I had to focus only on healing myself and not to get caught up in it," she stated. She thought that her Occupational Therapy sessions for the rehabilitation of her injured arm and hand were very therapeutic in many ways. She started with her bedside therapist whom she recalled; "I became attached to him because he was the first person to begin to heal me. He made an outrigger splint for me. He was very talkative and lovable. He even made a figurine for me out of the splinting material." She exhibits this figurine on her fireplace. When she transferred to the Hospital of Special Surgery for her hand therapy and follow-up surgeries, she recalled her interactions with the occupational therapists. She observed that the therapists were traumatized themselves. Many of the other clients would ask her about her injuries, so she would repeat her story. Some of the therapists would warn the others not to ask too many questions, but Judy believed that by sharing her story with the others it would be helpful for her to overcome her anxieties. She stated, "When people told their stories it affected me in a positive way because they would come together to help me understand how I felt when I saw the building coming down." She said that hearing other people's stories took her mind off her own issues and that she enjoyed their conversations. She thought that her therapists and environment were very supportive. Many times the therapists would discuss their own lives to keep her attention off of her own emotional problems. She said that by having physical injuries, she was able to divert her attention onto the rehabilitation and not onto the emotional anxiety she was experiencing.

Judy has used her experience to help others. "I thought if it makes others feel better then I would share my story and talk about it." Judy has helped surviving spouses find closure. Many wives of victims contacted her and asked if she had seen their husbands. Judy aided these women in the search for their husbands. She feels that this was an outlet for her. Judy has also set goals for herself. She has become more involved in restorative yoga, which she feels gives her peace and is a great release for her. She currently holds a small restorative yoga class for four older adults, three women and one man, in her home. "I think that they may feel sorry for me, and this is their way of comforting me," she chuckles.

Judy began working in November of 2001 from her home. She thought that by working at home, it would be easier to work around her therapy sessions. She has not returned to the city to work since the tragedy, but does venture in for important meetings. She had her home workstation ergonomically arranged to accommodate her injuries.

REFERENCE

Wein, J. & Rhodes, C. (2001, December). The Survivor from the 103rd Floor. *Ladies' Home Journal*, pp. 82-84. Used with permission.

Disabled and Experiencing Disaster: Personal and Professional Accounts

Hanna Diamond, MA, OTR
Pat Precin, MS, OTR/L

It was a beautiful Indian summer morning on Tuesday, September 11th. I was waiting for the M15 bus on the corner of 23rd Street and 1st Avenue on my way uptown to a New York City Hospital psychiatric day program. It was 8:30 a.m. I was beginning the fifth week of a 6-week per diem job as an occupational therapist and had already developed a comfortable morning routine. I got off at my stop, bought my morning coffee, walked to the clinic and took the elevator to the 13th floor. I had to lead the first group.

The building lobby was quiet. I entered the elevator with another woman and a man. The woman turned to me and said something very odd: "I just saw a plane hit the World Trade Tower. I was on the bridge coming into Manhattan when a plane hit the building." I felt goose bumps all over my skin as I replied "What?" She got off at her floor. I looked at the man; he showed no reaction.

As soon as the elevator door opened on my floor, I walked briskly down the hall. I needed more information. I had to find either a radio or a computer with Internet access. I needed to know more about this story. As I walked down the hallway, I looked out the windows. The beautiful blue sky did not have a cloud in it. I started to shake. I had a bad feeling about this day.

[Haworth co-indexing entry note]: "Disabled and Experiencing Disaster: Personal and Professional Accounts" Diamond, Hanna, and Pat Precin. Co-published simultaneously in *Occupational Therapy in Mental Health* (The Haworth Press, Inc.) Vol. 19, No. 3/4, 2003, pp. 27-41; and: *Surviving 9/11: Impact and Experiences of Occupational Therapy Practitioners* (ed: Pat Precin) The Haworth Press, Inc., 2003, pp. 27-41. Single or multiple copies of this article are available for a fee from The Haworth Document Delivery Service [1-800-HAWORTH, 9:00 a.m. - 5:00 p.m. (EST). E-mail address: docdelivery@haworthpress.com].

"Quick, turn on the radio," I called out to the staff. "A plane hit the World Trade Center!"

Someone replied, "I am sure it was just an accident. It was a small plane that hit the World Trade Center."

"No," I replied. "This is something else, something big, something bad." I thought, *I need to get home. I need to be with my family.*

A handful of clients had made it to the clinic program before the chaos in the city set in. I was instructed to begin the program for the day to provide structure and stability for the clientele who did make it in. I was a wreck, on the verge of tears. *I want to get home,* I thought. I began the morning group; the topic was anger management, but we wanted to talk about the World Trade Center. All of the clients in the group wanted to listen to the news. We found a radio and listened to conflicting news reports, trying to process what we heard. The Pentagon was hit. A second plane hit the second World Trade Tower. We turned off the radio and discussed our reactions until the end of the group session.

I ran to the phone and called my husband. "Honey, I am okay. Keep the children home. What about my niece, Jamie? Have you heard from her? She works in Tower One."

My husband replied, "A plane went down in Pennsylvania. Jamie made it out of Tower One and she is all right."

Looking out of the 13th floor window of the hospital clinic, I could see the 59th Street Bridge. Earlier, the only visible sign that something terribly wrong had happened was an ecru colored smoke plume streaming from behind the bridge towards Brooklyn. By noon, there was a mass of walkers making their way out of Manhattan towards Queens. In between the groups, clients and staff tried to get more information about the attack. Some clients were visibly shaken by the day's event; others were unusually calm and seemingly unaffected.

It was about 1:00 p.m. when we got word from administration that we could go home. Staff members were to assist clients home. This was organized by destination. Since I lived downtown, I was to help a group of seven clients reach their downtown destination. Our first goal was to get to the bus stop. Some clients did not feel capable of walking home. One complained of a bad back and an inability to walk any great distance. Others were very anxious. We had no choice but to begin our walk. A lot of people were walking north. There were no cars, except emergency vehicles. One of the staff members bumped into a friend of his who had been working at one of the towers. Luckily, he and his wife, who also worked at the World Trade Center, were safe. His friend was in shock and spoke about how he needed to find employment now that there was no income in the family. Second Avenue was chaotic. Police vehicles, sand trucks, unmarked cars and buses were moving south but many, many more people were walking north. Sirens were blaring.

Three buses were at the bus stop when we finally arrived. "If you cannot get on a bus, try the next," I told the clients. Five clients were able to get on the bus. A second staff member and I decided to walk with our remaining two clients. We had trouble moving through the northbound walkers. The 59th Street intersection was clogged with people and vehicles. We got separated. At 57th Street, I decided to get on a bus, but it sat motionless for a long time. People on the bus were quiet. Some kept trying their cell phones, but to no avail.

I could not tolerate the waiting so I got off the bus. On 55th Street, I ran into two clients who were told to get off the bus at 61st Street when the police took over their bus. We walked to 48th Street where together we waited for another bus.

It was then that I realized the streets were empty with only police cars moving south. Buses and sand trucks blocked the side streets leading to the United Nations building. After leaving the clients, I walked in the street because it was too difficult to dodge the crowd marching north. People were quiet. The city had an eerie silence to it. Some people were walking barefoot.

Two hours later I finally reached 23rd Street where there was a lot of police activity. The Police Academy was located on 20th Street between 2nd Avenue and 3rd Avenue, and had large police vans blocking the entrance to the street. I did not know it then, but this was the Mayor's command center.

I made it to 20th Street and 1st Avenue. It was a sea of traffic. Cars were heading north. This was an emergency conduit from the Downtown area to Bellevue and the New York University Hospitals. Twentieth Street east of 1st Avenue towards the Franklin D. Roosevelt (FDR) Highway was closed except for rescue vehicles.

I walked towards the FDR highway to my apartment, saw my husband, my children and niece and started to cry. My four-year-old son hid in the closet before asking me why I was crying. I later found out that he had watched the planes hit the towers over and over the entire day as neighbors and family members congregated at my apartment to hear and watch the events going on downtown. He thought that each time there was a replay of a tower being hit that it was a new building and a new plane. In his mind, his home was being destroyed building by building.

Somehow, I had been able to walk home in spite of having severe rheumatoid arthritis. I have been limping over the last few years because of the pain I experience. On that day, I suffered no physical pain. I had not eaten, but was not hungry. I was scared. I was worried. My niece had been on the 32nd floor of Tower One when the plane struck Tower Two. She said she saw office equipment fly past her window. Her supervisor told the office to evacuate. She was near Century 21 when Tower One, her tower, was hit. In her confusion, she somehow made it to our apartment.

That first night was quiet and eerie. My niece asked that I sleep with her. In the morning, she told me that she had not slept. She swore that she heard the fighter planes taking off and landing on the navy carrier located outside of the New York harbor and that the sounds of the rescue vehicles kept her awake all night. I did not sleep well, but I heard nothing.

The next few days I was very irritable. The sounds of the fighter planes overhead unnerved me; the smell of the smoke sickened me, and seeing the missing-people posters agitated me. I panicked when I saw the plume of a large fire from the local Con Edison plant. The makeshift memorials appeared everywhere. A quiet, depressive aura covered New York City (Photos 1-3).

I did some reading in order to decrease my anxiety and apprehension. I learned that regular memories and trauma memories are encoded differently. Regular memories are encoded predominantly through language while trauma memories are deeply encoded on a non-verbal sensory level. Now I understand why I was not hungry during that day, and why I was not feeling the degree of physical pain I am used to experiencing. I understand why I had such strong emotional reactions to sensory stimuli.

I thought about my experience on September 11th at the day program, i.e., how well the psychiatric clients seemed to manage during this crisis. They were calm and wanted to talk about the situation. Everyone supported each other throughout the day and on the journey home. No one became psychotic. In fact, some were more worried about the staff than themselves. There seemed to have been a flight into health. This further confirmed my belief regarding the mentally ill and their ability to cope with stress. I have twenty-plus years experience of working with individuals with mental illness. Often I have felt that it is the daily hassles that are hard for many to cope with, and that there is strength in many of these individuals to cope with major life stressors, such as homelessness, and death.

PHOTO 1. Ash Covered Cars.

Photo by Gilad Rosner. Used by permission.

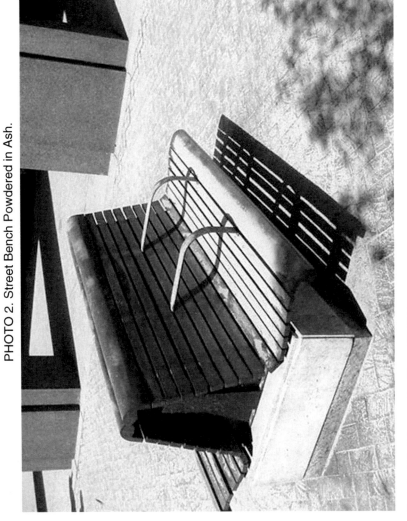

PHOTO 2. Street Bench Powdered in Ash.

Photo by Gilad Rosner. Used by permission.

PHOTO 3. Burnt Paper.

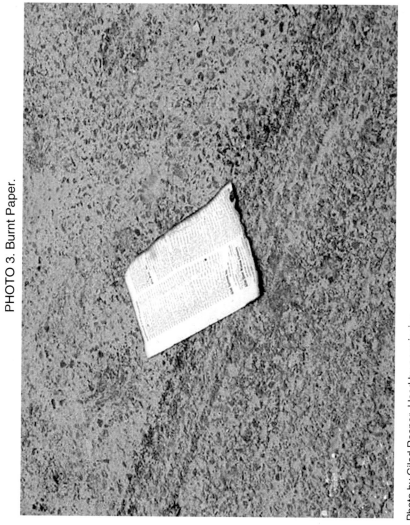

33

Having returned home safely, secured the safety of my family, seen to it that my clients were all right, done some research and reflected on the whole experience, I began to be less anxious and more centered. Having a physical disability myself (rheumatoid arthritis) and having helped a group of psychiatric clients suffering from schizophrenia, depression, and bipolar illness find their way home to safety amidst the chaos and turmoil just described, made me very sensitive to disabled people's needs in time of disaster. I knew I wanted to help other disabled people manage the aftermath of September 11th and prepare for another possible emergency. I had an opportunity to attend a Federal Emergency Management Agency (FEMA)/Center for Mental Health Services (CMHS) Crises Counseling Assistance and Training Program through my job. I was one of many social service workers there. During this one-day training, I was introduced to how FEMA organizes several federal agencies to work on a local level to provide disaster relief on an economic, spiritual, and emotional level. The Center for Mental Health Services partnered with the Office for Victims of Crime, The National Center on Post-Traumatic Stress Disorders, The National Transportation Service Board, the National Institute of Mental Health and the United States Department of Education to form the 9/11 disaster relief program called Project Liberty to meet the needs of the people of New York.

"No one who sees a disaster is untouched by it" (DeWolfe, 2000). Through Project Liberty, contacts among the various social agencies were fostered in order to develop a comprehensive program to address the psychosocial needs of physically disabled people in their homes, among circles of friends and family, and during their daily activities. I would be going to disabled housing, i.e., single-room occupancies (SROs) designed for people who are physically disabled. I would provide a general introduction to available disaster relief services, a description of the normal response to trauma, and an introduction to stress management techniques. I was now a Project Liberty worker.

During the six-hour FEMA/CMHS training, I learned the differences between traditional mental health counseling and disaster mental health counseling. Unlike traditional mental health counseling, people seeking help would not be labeled by a diagnosis, would not receive case management services, and would not be seen in an office. Rather, they were to be contacted and seen in their communities. I was to listen to people's experiences, validate the appropriateness of their reactions, educate them about normal responses to trauma, encourage the use of available disaster relief services, uncover previous styles of dealing with stress, promote the use of coping skills and adaptations that worked in the past, encourage the return to a pre-disaster typical daily routine, help the person identify a high priority problem, and then develop and implement a plan. If I thought a person needed more than crisis counseling, I was to refer him/her to available traditional mental health services.

I also learned that trauma is experienced on a collective level as well as an individual level. Immediately after the disaster, there is a heroic phase–to assist in the recovery phase. This is followed by a honeymoon period in which the community works together. As time goes on there is disillusionment. The community needs to come to terms with the disruption of existing social and community patterns and must work through grief before reconstructing a new beginning. This last phase can take years, as was the case in the Oklahoma City disaster, to which people are still reacting five years later.

From my FEMA education, I was able to set up a two-hour psycho-educational program designed to educate people about available disaster relief programs, to describe normal reactions to trauma, and to promote adequate stress management. I also added a piece about emergency preparedness for those with a disability, for I felt that this warranted a special focus.

I had been sent to two disabled-housing programs that housed residents with either a physical and/or a psychiatric disability. My first presentation was formal, as the residents had difficulty participating in the discussions. Instead of being able to talk about their individual reactions to 9/11, they were more focused on their long-standing individual problems that existed prior to 9/11. The second group I met with had already been able to mobilize a response to 9/11 by making food for the local police and fire departments, and presenting them with trophies for their heroic work. This group initially stated that they were not interested in Project Liberty but had agreed to meet with me for twenty minutes; we met for two hours. Many of the men were angry and wanted to discuss the United States' response to the bombing. Eventually, people spoke about their reactions. One woman spoke about her difficulty in going back to her routine, as she was scared. "I do not know if I could get back to church, something might happen," she said. Others had watched from their rooms as the towers fell. They got upset when viewing the new skyline void of the buildings that once stood. One was worried for her child who had been exposed to the trauma. She did not know how to respond to her child. One was afraid to go outdoors since the smoke would aggravate an existing respiratory problem.

I also had the opportunity to do an individual counseling session in a woman's home. She was an intelligent, driven woman who in the past had traveled to the Third World to help people in need. She had developed a chronic fatigue illness a few years earlier and was now feeling devastated by 9/11. She was angry that she could not be of more assistance downtown, but she had nightmares, and flinched each time she heard a plane overhead. She ran down to Union Square at all hours of the night to participate in the memorial rituals. She stated, "My friends are tired of hearing me talk about 9/11."

All of the reactions mentioned above are typical reactions to a disaster. Other normal behavioral reactions to a disaster include sleep disturbances. My husband could not sleep after 9/11; he was on alert to keep his family safe and to be able to act quickly if there was any trouble. Crying easily, angry outbursts, and greater family conflicts are additional normal responses. I cried every time I saw a missing persons' poster (Photo 4) or walked past the "Wall of Prayer." The "Wall of Prayer" was created on a wooden construction wall that lined the walkway into Bellevue Hospital. It was decorated with missing persons' posters, prayers, drawings and memorials. Each day it grew; each day I cried. I was also very short tempered and remember that I yelled at my kids more easily. Hypervigilance and startle reactions are also expected. Many of my friends were very aware of airplanes after 9/11 and would freeze if one seemed unusually low. Others expressed concern that an increase in helicopter air congestion was surely indicative of trouble. Other behavioral reactions include higher activity levels with lower productivity, withdrawal and isolation manifested by reluctance to leave home, an avoidance of reminders, and increased use of drugs, alcohol, sugar, nicotine, and caffeine.

Physical reactions to trauma include feelings of fatigue and exhaustion (many of my co-workers described feeling overly-tired), stomach and digestive problems (my supervisor developed a severe gastrointestinal problem during the week following 9/11), headaches and other pains, colds and flu symptoms, and worsening of health problems (another friend of mine developed the shingles).

The cognitive manifestations following a disaster include repetitive worries and thoughts, difficulty concentrating, difficulty making plans and decisions, limited attention span, and memory problems. The cognitive reactions can be further compounded by emotions such as feeling hopeless, helpless, anxious, irritable, angry, depressed, guilty, and/or

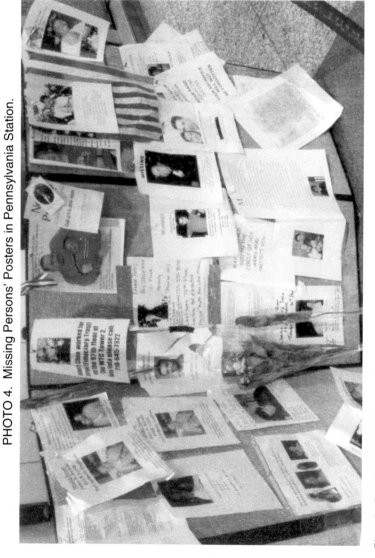

PHOTO 4. Missing Persons' Posters in Pennsylvania Station.

Photo by Fran Babiss. Used by permission.

ashamed. Some of my clients asked, "How could this have happened? What can I do to help? I feel so useless. Will this happen again?"

If the above-described reactions to a disaster are considered normal, then what is the impact on those with disabilities? People with disabilities need additional time to evacuate. Their ability to process information may be impeded because of auditory, visual, sensory, mobility or cognitive impairments. They are more physically vulnerable from prior chronic health conditions. People with impaired mobility descend stairs slowly if at all. They may be afraid of being lifted for fear of being dropped in a chaotic situation. People with cognitive deficits may become further confused or disoriented about how to react in an emergency. A deaf or hard-of-hearing person may not be able to hear or understand the warning and emergency instructions. A blind or visually impaired person may be reluctant to leave familiar surroundings even if the surroundings are not safe. Healthy bodied individuals were scared and confused. Can you imagine what it would be like to be slowed by a disability and not be able to reach safety? (The Elk's Camp Moore and Special Olympics children can, and they showed their appreciation for differently abled people and the rescuers that helped them by creating the memorial banner in Photo 5 and signing their t-shirts as in Photo 6 all of which hang near Ground Zero).

In addition to evacuation needs, there are other concerns. What are the individual's medication needs? Does he/she have extra medications available? Those on strict medication regimes may become concerned about having medications suddenly stopped. Who is aware of the person's medication schedule, dosages, and pharmacy? Is it advisable to encourage clients to skim off a few pills a week so that an extra week's worth of medication is available if needed? Or can the individual get a special prescription from the doctor for a separate emergency supply of medications? What if a person takes medication that is a controlled substance? How will he/she get an emergency supply?

There are other difficulties faced by those with disabilities. There can be a loss of home health support, a significant problem. Can the home health aid travel to get to the client? In addition, the isolation that is common for individuals with disabilities may further compound the lack of awareness of disaster-related resources. Lack of transportation and limited mobility may make it harder for an individual to get to disaster-relief sites. As a result, individuals with disabilities tend to under-utilize disaster-relief services.

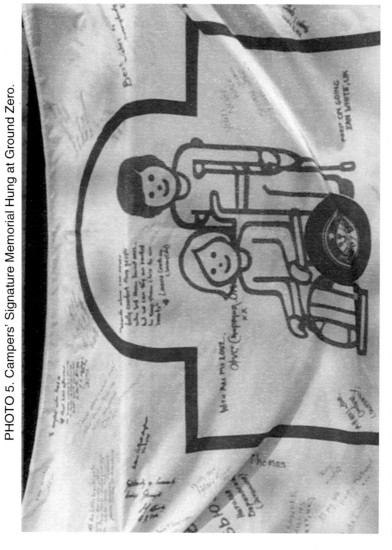

PHOTO 5. Campers' Signature Memorial Hung at Ground Zero.

Photo by Pat Precin. Used by permission.

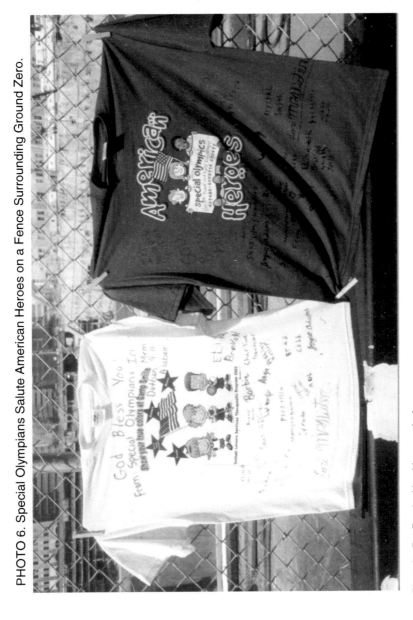

PHOTO 6. Special Olympians Salute American Heroes on a Fence Surrounding Ground Zero.

Photo by Pat Precin. Used by permission.

Interventions for people with disabilities include stress management, empowering techniques, emergency plans, and crisis counseling. Stress management and empowerment techniques for disaster counseling for a general population include discussing reactions; maintaining a typical daily routine; spending time with friends, loved ones, and family members; using pre-disaster existing support groups; participating in rituals or memorials; trying not to feel frustrated about not being able to help directly; maintaining a healthy diet; and avoiding unhealthy coping styles. In addition, people with disabilities require an emergency plan. This emergency plan may include but is not limited to: a buddy system; a week's worth of medications; and extra equipment such as walkers, wheelchairs, eyeglasses, hearing aids with fresh batteries, and/or generators to maintain oxygen supplies. It is because the needs of individuals with disabilities are so varied that the development of a self-help network is encouraged.

LIFENET recently extended their financial coverage up to one year for the treatment of psychological issues related to 9/11. LIFENET phone lines are available 24 hours a day to refer people to a Project Liberty center. The English-speaking phone line is 1-800-LIFENET. The Spanish-speaking phone line is 1-877-AYUDESE. The Chinese-speaking phone line is ASIAN LIFENET. Further information regarding crisis mental health can be obtained via the Web at *http://www.mentalhealth.org* and *http://www.fema.gov*

REFERENCE

DeWolfe, D.J. (2000). *The field manual for mental health and human service workers in major disasters: Key concepts of disaster mental health.* Washington, D.C.: National Mental Health Services Knowledge Exchange Network.

Being There

Mary V. Donohue, PhD, OT, FAOTA

It was a perfectly beautiful fall day, with stillness in the air that engenders a feeling of the Garden of Eden, and a wish that would preserve the day forever. My Long Island Railroad train was just about to enter the tunnel under the East River at 8:55 a.m. when the conductor announced: "There is a fire in one of the Trade Towers. You had better check to see if your subway is running." I decided to walk from Pennsylvania Station, at 34th Street, to New York University, Department of Occupational Therapy, on West 4th Street, near Washington Square Park, so as not to get stuck in a subway. As I headed south, I wondered if I should go back home, but continued onward, thinking about being with the New York University occupational therapy faculty, rather than being alone at home. As I walked along 7th Avenue, I could see the smoke billowing upward (Photo 1). This was not a small fire. The avenue was filled with people standing out in the middle of the street and watching the smoke in disbelief (Photo 2). Fire trucks were passing southward filled with firefighters hanging on the outside, and I worried for them as to how they could handle a towering inferno.

After walking southward for about ten minutes, I decided to turn eastward to Broadway, to continue towards New York University. As I came to Broadway and 22nd Street people were screaming, "I just saw another plane crash into the other Trade Tower." I said to one person, "World War III." I thought about how frightened I was as a child during World War II when there were blackout practices and enemy subma-

---

[Haworth co-indexing entry note]: "Being There." Donohue, Mary V. Co-published simultaneously in *Occupational Therapy in Mental Health* (The Haworth Press, Inc.) Vol. 19, No. 3/4, 2003, pp. 43-50; and: *Surviving 9/11: Impact and Experiences of Occupational Therapy Practitioners* (ed: Pat Precin) The Haworth Press, Inc., 2003, pp. 43-50. Single or multiple copies of this article are available for a fee from The Haworth Document Delivery Service [1-800-HAWORTH, 9:00 a.m. - 5:00 p.m. (EST). E-mail address: docdelivery@haworthpress.com].

Digital Object Identifier: 10.1300/J004v19n03_04

PHOTO 1. Smoke Billowing Upward.

Photo by Gilad Rosner. Used by permission.

44

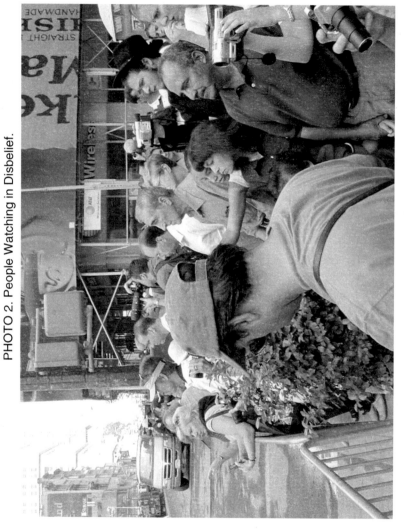

PHOTO 2. People Watching in Disbelief.

Photo by Donna Brennan. Used by permission.

rines off Long Island. More fire trucks were passing southward toward the Towers, and I continued to fear for the lives of those men, moving toward the destruction.

I always loved looking at the skyline of New York as I crossed the Throgs Neck Bridge by car, in particular the most identifiable buildings, the Towers, Empire State, Chrysler, Metropolitan Life Insurance, and Citicorp, all a part of the Big Apple; but simultaneously, as I felt a surge of admiration, I had a second sad thought, that the World Trade Center was a target. After the 1993 terror attack on the Trade Towers, the terrorists promised to return, and they did.

From the 11th floor of the Education Building of New York University, the occupational therapy faculty, students, and I watched the towers of smoke blowing north, hiding the skyscrapers. We asked each other if the towers were still there, and then saw on television that they had collapsed.

We sent one class of students home, asking them first if they had known anyone who worked at the World Trade Center. Two second-year students were worried sick. One had a brother and the other a twin sister with jobs there. Cell phone communication was knocked out when the towers went down, but the twin shortly called her family to say that she was all right. The brother had gone out for coffee as the planes struck. He jumped into his van, taking people with him, but could not find a phone without a line-up of people waiting to use it until well into the evening. Nor could he find a bridge to cross out of Manhattan that was not streaming with people walking to Queens and Brooklyn. Our student had gone home to console her mother during those terrible hours of waiting. Ultimately, we were relieved that none of our students had lost any family or close friends.

In between classes, students and faculty listened and watched the news on the television that we placed in our largest lab. How many planes were still in the sky? Where were they?

We let students from out of state call home. Their parents wanted them to leave New York, but there was no way to do so.

New York University wished to remain open, especially because the semester had just begun, and out-of-town students wanted to begin the semester to keep busy given what was happening, especially if it was their first semester away from home. Starting school helped some of these students take their minds off the disaster and kept them from feeling helpless in a new setting. My teaching partner's lecture material for the next day was stuck in her apartment near the Trade Towers. She knew that she could not go home, so I stayed late to help her prepare a class to present.

The New York University had dorms near the Towers. The dorms had to be evacuated and students were brought to the Coles' Student Center, then relocated to hotels. Later that night, I saw from an e-mail message that Mayor Giuliani closed every enterprise south of 14th Street to all but emergency personnel. As I walked to the subway, the streets were desolate, with barely a moving vehicle. Manhattan was a ghost town.

The New York University's Home Network alerted us not to come to work the next day, Wednesday. However, on Wednesday evening, the School of Education asked that any faculty with mental health experience report to work on Thursday to help counsel students. We were told to show identification at 14th Street; however, at 14th Street, our identifications were not requested, and the subway continued on to West 4th Street. First, faculty had a briefing by a university psychologist on post-traumatic stress disorder. We were given a handout with a list of symptoms, beginning with the inability to concentrate, a symptom that can plague students. I made copies for our faculty and students to put in their mailboxes.

Our dean had set up a pizza party for all students from the school who wished to come to speak to faculty about their concerns. I spent time with one student who was from Washington, District of Columbia, and who was to return there that weekend for a wedding. She felt like she was going from the frying pan into the fire, going from New York, at this time, to Washington, District of Columbia, and she dreaded going to stay with her parents, because she felt that she could not talk to them about her feelings. "They always suppressed everything," she bemoaned. After listening and thinking about it, I said to her, "Tell your parents that the dean had a pizza party so people could talk about feelings, and tell them about our conversation together, so they will see how we valued feelings at New York University."

I approached another group of students sitting together. They were all from Canada, and feeling very lost in the emotional upheaval of the event, not being American, but frightened, nonetheless. One was tearful, saying that she is a Muslim, and she was afraid of how people were going to treat her, despite the fact that she was really French with French citizenship. In this case, I thought it best to be concrete. I said to her, "Tell people that you are French." I thought that this would give them pause to check their biases, and perhaps review their reactions. I also wished to remind her that she was more than her religion.

By this time, almost all the students who attended the counseling session/pizza party in Pless Hall, overlooking Washington Square Park, had spoken to some faculty. I was glad for that, because I suddenly felt emotionally overwhelmed myself. There are many unexpected issues associated with the terror attacks. I was glad to go out to lunch with a fellow faculty so that we could support each other. I recalled what one of our associate deans had said to us on our way out: "Take care of yourselves, too."

HOW DO I FEEL NOW?

Am I ever fearful of traveling from the suburbs into New York City? Yes, especially on the subways, which could be the target of microbial, viral or chemical attacks, and which have a very poor public announcement system. In the event of such an attack, clear communications would be needed to keep the public informed. I also fear being downwind of a possible attack on the Indian Point atomic energy plant located in Westchester, New York. And on beautiful, clear days, with perfectly still skies, I think that it was just like this when. . . . What a terrible association to have with amazingly blue skies that can no longer be dreamy for me.

Weeks and weeks of reading biographies of victims in the newspaper enlightened me on the individuality of the people who had died. They were lively people working in a vital space and now they are gone. They became personally known through their photographs and stories of activities that they liked to engage in during their lives. These stories were very occupation-oriented. Many of the victims who had worked in the World Trade Center Towers as support workers or careered employees had resided in Long Island. Family and other Long Islanders sorely miss their presence, and multitudinous memorials have appeared throughout the Island.

The psychological landscape of my perspective has changed. The possibility of sleeper cells waiting to attack, still hating our lifestyle, our civilization, our city is always there as a backdrop on the stage of our New World. Yet, the New World has more focus, more love and more cohesion among people of the metropolitan area. We are still aware that many neighbors, colleagues and family can be suffering from the shock of seeing the impact of the planes, the post-traumatic stress of survival, watching the devastation on television, emotions stirred on visiting Ground Zero, general anxiety that haunts memories, and from depression, acknowledged or unacknowledged.

As part of my own response, I have designed a Ground Zero Memorial, a meditation arena with wooden or stone seats in concentric circles, and submitted it to the architects and planners of the Lower Manhattan Redevelopment Project (see Figure 1). The suggested inscription reads: *"In memory of all who died here in 1993 and 2001. May our enemies become our friends."*

FIGURE 1. Ground Zero Memorial by Mary Donohue

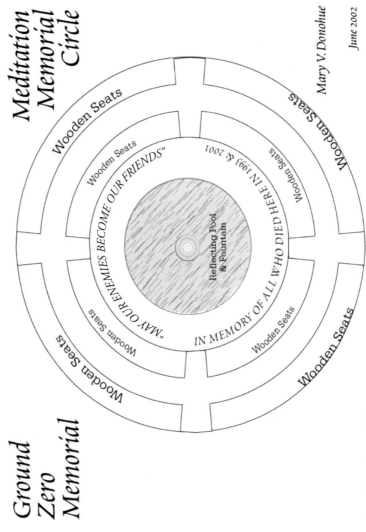

Meditation
Memorial
Circle

Ground
Zero
Memorial

Wooden Seats

Wooden Seats

Wooden Seats

Wooden Seats

Wooden Seats

Wooden Seats

Wooden Seats

Wooden Seats

Wooden Seats

"MAY OUR ENEMIES BECOME OUR FRIENDS"

IN MEMORY OF ALL WHO DIED HERE IN 1993 & 2001

Reflecting Pool & Fountain

Mary V. Donohue

June 2002

Graphics: Fran Babiss

9/11:
A Muslim Occupational Therapy Student's Perspective

Sabina Luna, OTS

Diane B. Tewfik, MA, OTR/L

I was in the 8:00 a.m. class on the day of September 11. During my break, I made a phone call to my husband who told me that a plane had just crashed into the Twin Towers and that a few thousand people were supposed dead. I immediately returned to my class and told some of my classmates that there had been a terrible accident. We all rushed to the Occupational Therapy Department office and found through the Internet that it was a possible terrorist attack, not an accident. I remember trembling in fear as I thought of the possibility that a Muslim may have committed this act. I am Muslim and I worried about the future consequences of this act towards our religion and people.

I remembered the situation after the Oklahoma bombing when many Muslims were being questioned. My first concern was to make sure my husband and son arrived home safely. I was especially worried because they have typical Muslim names. My son attends high school in Manhattan and has to travel a long way by subway. I tried to call my husband, but the cell-phone was dead. After a few trials from my professor's office telephone at York College, I reached him and learned that he was going to pick up my son. I remember that a few other stu-

---

[Haworth co-indexing entry note]: "9/11: A Muslim Occupational Therapy Student's Perspective." Luna, Sabina, and Diane B. Tewfik. Co-published simultaneously in *Occupational Therapy in Mental Health* (The Haworth Press, Inc.) Vol. 19, No. 3/4, 2003, pp. 51-58; and: *Surviving 9/11: Impact and Experiences of Occupational Therapy Practitioners* (ed: Pat Precin) The Haworth Press, Inc., 2003, pp. 51-58. Single or multiple copies of this article are available for a fee from The Haworth Document Delivery Service [1-800-HAWORTH, 9:00 a.m. - 5:00 p.m. (EST). E-mail address: docdelivery@haworthpress.com].

Digital Object Identifier: 10.1300/J004v19n03_05

dents were crying along with me. When I started weeping, the professors and my classmates were very supportive.

I left school and headed for the bus. My seventy-nine-year-old mother was at home. She is diabetic. My concern was that someone might call home to inform her of the attacks and that her resultant anxiety may create a health condition for her. The people on the street seemed alarmed. I stopped by my 6-year-old daughter's school to pick her up. Hundreds of parents rushed to school to pick up their children. I remember a school official approached me and advised me not to look so worried in front of my daughter.

I felt relieved, discovering my mother drying her laundry in the sun when I got home. She complained that something happened to the television sets. They were not working. She said that a few people had called and asked for me. I told my mom about the incident. She expressed concern about her grandson and my husband. Although she looked surprised, having grown up and lived in a place where terrorism is a daily routine, my mother seemed immune to this kind of news. After saying one or two words about the situation, she went away to do her daily errands. I hid a sad smile when my mother expressed disappointment toward me that I did not bring "Hilsa" fish, which goes best with the young pumpkin she grew in my backyard.

I sat down on the sofa and witnessed the terrible scenes on the television. Time was passing and I was worried and anxious. I realized that nothing was more important to me than having my family around me. I did not have any appetite. My husband and my son arrived home around 11:00 p.m. They had walked across the Queens Bridge.

Within a few days, we started to hear about scattered incidents towards Muslims. My nephew's friend, Yusuf, arrived home to find that his house gate had been destroyed by some neighborhood men who had posted a note saying, "Go back to your country." Astoria is known as "little Bangladesh." Most incidents I heard about happened in that area. Even though there were incidents among other Muslim communities, I can talk about only my own community, the Bangladeshi people. A few Bangladeshi people were mugged and they were addressed as "F–king Muslims," even though one of them was Hindu. I heard that a covered-lady was beaten. We talked with friends and family, and everyone had a story to tell about the harassment of suspected Muslims.

All the people I knew who had mothers living with them insisted that their mothers not "cover" themselves when they went out. My mother also covers her head and wears modest clothing (not a burkha or chador that most people think Muslim women wear), but I could not or did not want to forbid her to do that. I felt sorry and violated. It was her culture and a lifelong practice she grew up with. I could not ask her to abandon her belief system because of some misinformed and ignorant people. My mother is a very smart and intelligent woman, whose hobbies are reading and watching historical and science-fiction movies. She sensed our tension and anxiety when we went out. Every time we wanted to go out, my mom started to make an excuse for staying home. She knows that I do not live according to other people's expectations.

I am the revolutionary in the family. I am the first one in the family who had a love-marriage. All of my eight brothers and sisters had arranged marriages. I am the one who wears Western outfits. She knew that I would never allow her to stay home because she was scared of being harassed as a Muslim woman. Nor would I ask her to leave her shawl. But I compromised anyway. I encouraged my mom to walk around my backyard and not to go out to the neighborhood. I completely stopped wearing "shalware-kameej" (traditional South Asian dress). So did most of the women of my community. My mother sensed that we were extra-cautious because of her. She started to talk about going back to Bangladesh. She was supposed to stay until my graduation. She became depressed staying home. So, I let her go back to Bangladesh.

After my mother left, I began to feel depressed. My thinking process was changing. I am usually very realistic. I do not worry much. Even in an extremely troubling situation, I manage to stay cool and try to resolve the problem in a systematic way instead of panicking. *(I remember one situation back in 1988 in Bangladesh. I was teaching the alphabet to my 3-year-old son in the evening on my bed. Suddenly, a big explosion broke the glass of my windows. I picked up my son and went to another part of the house. We lived in a joint-family home. All of my in-laws were screaming. After I placed my son in a safe place, I went straight to the phone and called for help. In a corrupted country like Bangladesh, there are no 911 numbers to call, nor will the police always help. I called just the right person who could help us. It was a cocktail bomb thrown by a moving car toward a building next to ours. The building was the office of a weekly magazine, where they recently published something against Muslim Fundamentalists. Everybody in the family was surprised that I was acting like a robot instead of responding emotionally.)*

I started my psychosocial fieldwork level 1 during the first week of September. My supervisor was a Japanese-American who was in her sixties. I called my supervisor right after the incident and found out that everything was all right with them. On my next day of the fieldwork, I found that the therapists were offering counseling service to people who were affected by the incident. Naturally, we talked about the tragedy. My supervisor asked me if I had to face any trouble because of the situation. I did not tell her that I was Muslim or where had I come from. Yet she was most confident in her guess of my identity. We are not similar to the people suspected of this incident, physically, culturally, or geographically. Her inquiry was an eye-opener for me. I thought most people knew that Indians are Hindu. Everyone in my family looks like Indians. I never thought that I could be seen differently. I became more anxious for my son's safety. He has to take a long ride to school every day. He is very proud of being a Muslim and a Bangladeshi-American.

My anxiety increased to a panic state after a conversation with my fieldwork supervisor. She told me that after the Pearl Harbor bombing, all the people of Japanese descent were taken to concentration camps, even though they were American citizens. She said that afterward her brother joined the United States Army just to prove patriotism of a Japanese-American. She thought the same thing could happen to Muslims, too. I had no knowledge about those concentration camps. I read about the concentration camps during the Holocaust. I could not imagine that there could be concentration camps in America. Those thoughts and some other scattered incidents slowly started to disrupt my daily life. I heard that one of our relatives was asked to disembark the plane when he was traveling from Los Angeles to New York. He was an American by birth. Although he has a Muslim name and dark skin, he knew and followed very little of the Muslim religion. After a long interrogation, he was allowed to board, but the pilot refused to fly if he was on the plane. This kind of harassment was both insulting and frightening to all of us.

I did not realize that I was becoming more and more depressed until I had Psychosocial Occupational Therapy class, where I learned that my excessive eating, excessive sleeping, and unwillingness to talk to others were all symptoms. I felt very bad that my mother had left the country. My father died two years ago, so my mother lives alone back home. My husband becomes nervous very easily. He has hypertension, which runs in his family. I never discuss stressful situations with him. Now, he was constantly worried about our son even though we gave our son a cell-phone to use in an emergency.

Even though I have a few good friends, I did not talk about my feelings. I did not realize or maybe did not want to admit or believe that I could be going through a situation that required help from someone else. I tried to study, but I could not concentrate. I applied all the techniques to increase concentration and relieve stress that I learned from my Collaboration in Occupational Therapy class, but none of them worked. I could not remember the formal definitions of terms. My head felt very heavy. When it lasted over a week, my husband forced me to go to the doctor. I found out that my blood pressure was very high. It was so high that he gave me medication to control it. I always have normal blood pressure. My family does not have a history of high blood pressure. I could not remember one term or definition asked on the midterm exam.

Graduating in the occupational therapy program is the most important task of my life. Not only I, but also my entire family is devoted to my receiving this degree. I take my studies very seriously. I already lost so many years of academic achievement because of an early marriage and motherhood. Studying was the most important job for me now, but all my hard work was in vain. I simply could not remember. At that time, I thought I was having bad luck, even though I do not believe in luck. But when my ability to concentrate continued to be poor, I started to ask myself, *What is going on? Why can I not concentrate?* I did not want to believe that I could be a victim of the situation. I am supposed to help the victim. That is what I used to do. I am very much appreciated by people for giving them support/advice when they need it. Now I am the one who cannot function fully because of the anxiety I feel in my surroundings.

There was no particular harassment that happened to my family or to me. It is the possibility of harassment that scares me. Muslims are not being hired for jobs. In this democratic country, the employers choose whom they want to hire and when employers see a Muslim name, they throw the application in the trashcan. This makes me nervous. I invested all my money towards my education. It is hard to concentrate when I think that I may not be hired because of my religion. In Bangladesh, there are many physical therapists, but occupational therapy does not exist.

My teachers at school started to sense that something was going wrong. Struggling with so many roles (mother, student, employee and wife), my performance was not perfect. Throughout the semester, I started to avoid any advising sessions. I practically hid myself from an approaching teacher in the hallway. I do not know what got into me. My advisor and the entire faculty in the Occupational Therapy Program are very approachable and available, yet I did not take the opportunity to talk to someone professional who could help me find a solution to my situation.

The most devastating issue of my situation was dealing with my studies. All the time I was wondering why I could not concentrate and remember. I started to sense that I was not all right when my grades dropped drastically. When I met with my professor, she told me that I should have come to her and together we could have found a solution to avoid my poor concentration and forgetfulness. She was right. All that time I was very sensitive and I was afraid I would start to cry when I talked. I knew that it was all right to cry, but my ego did not allow me to talk to the faculty about personal issues and feelings. It was not a wise decision.

Today Professor Tewfik asked me if I have gotten over my depression. I actually do not know. Writing about the situation surely helped me. At last, I expressed myself. I actually thought she tricked me into writing this by telling me this would be in a book and it would help others. I am still not comfortable talking about my feelings. I think the fear of being labeled as a 9/11 victim was the main issue for me in not identifying and admitting my depression. I also did not want people to approach me with pity and ask me if I was all right. But I could have avoided a lot of distress by talking to professionals.

* * *

You have just read the story of an occupational therapy student with the same course load, fieldwork requirements, enthusiasm, motivation and self-doubt as most occupational therapy students. However, she is from Bangladesh, a Muslim, an employee, a mother and a wife with a myriad of family responsibilities along with her occupational therapy schoolwork. Her story is about an occupational therapy student who also became a victim of 9/11 because of her religious and ethnic background. She was learning to help others, but needed to learn how to help herself first.

Much of the recent occupational therapy and other health-related professions' literature (see Bibliography) concerns how to help students and clinicians attain cultural competency, professional development, and critical reasoning to enhance client care. Occupational therapists sometimes fail to see that these concepts apply to themselves as well. Understanding that we as therapists can be stressed beyond our own limits and can also suffer from anxiety, depression, and Post-Traumatic Stress Disorder is one thing, but acknowledging it when it happens and asking for help is another. We also can have our own biases and our own prejudices, which can interfere not only with our effectively treating our patients, but also with our ability to be objective about our own behaviors. Being vulnerable to the same illnesses that our patients may have can be very upsetting to people, and denial is a common defense.

Students, because of their very demanding schedules, are concerned with learning facts and taking tests. Real life integration is a much more difficult process. The real challenge is to understand and use the essence of cultural competency and the therapeutic use of one's self. Besides learning about other people's cultures and beliefs, it is necessary to understand how and when our own cultures, our own beliefs and values are being threatened and how this affects our ability to help others. We need to develop support systems, listen to ourselves, seek counseling and talk about our feelings with people who can help. Self-awareness and cultural competency increase the ability to help others not just as occupational therapists but as human beings. With so much world strife, people need to be accountable for their actions and behaviors. People need to look at situations from different perspectives and understand that 9/11, the Holocaust, the atrocities in Sarajevo, the Japanese/American interment during the war, and all racial profiling should never have happened and should not reoccur. Self-examination can begin to make a difference.

SUGGESTED BIBLIOGRAPHY

Barbee, E. L. (1993). Racism in US nursing. *Medical Anthropology Quarterly*, 7(4), 346-362.

Black, R. M. (2002). Occupational therapy's dance with diversity. *The American Journal of Occupational Therapy*, 56, 140-148.

Bonder, B., Martin, L., & Miracle, A. (2002). *Culture in clinical care*. Thorofare, NJ: Slack, Inc.

Cena, L., McGruder, J., & Tomlin, G. (2002). Representations of race, ethnicity, and social class in case examples in *The American Journal of Occupational Therapy*. *The American Journal of Occupational Therapy*, 56, 130-139.

Cross, T. L., Bazron, B. J., Dennis, K. W., & Isaacs, M. R. (1989). *Towards a culturally competent system of care*, Volume 1. Washington, DC: CASSP Technical Assistance Center.

Dillard, M., Andonian, L., Flores, O., Lai, L., MacRae, A., & Shakir, M. (1992). Culturally competent occupational therapy in a diversely populated mental health setting. *American Journal of Occupational Therapy*, 46, 721-726.

Fadiman, A. (1997). *The spirit catches you and you fall down*. NY: Noonday Press.

Kleinman, A. (1980). *Patients and healers in the context of culture*. Berkeley: University of California Press.

Leavitt, R. L. (Ed.). (2001). *Cross-cultural rehabilitation: An international perspective*. Philadelphia: WB Saunders, Co.

Luckman, J., & Nobles, S.T. (2000). *Transcultural communication in health care.* United States: Delmar Thomson Learning.

Pope-Davis, D. B., Prietor, L. R., Whitaker, C. M., & Pope-Davis, S.A. (1993). Exploring multicultural competencies of occupational therapists: Implications for education and training. *The American Journal of Occupational Therapy, 47*, 838-844.

Spencer, J., Hersch, G., Shelton, M., Ripple, J., Spencer, C., Dryer, C. B., & Murphy, K. (2002). Functional outcomes and daily life activities of African-American elders after hospitalization. *The American Journal of Occupational Therapy, 56*, 149-159.

Wells, S. A., & Black, R. M. (2000). *Cultural competency for health professionals.* Bethesda, Maryland: The American Occupational Therapy Association, Inc.

Wittman, P., & Velde, B. P. (2002). *The Issue Is–Attaining cultural competence, critical thinking, and intellectual development: A challenge for occupational therapists, 56*, 454-456.

Personal Perspective on 9/11

Ann Burkhardt, MA, OTR/L, FAOTA, BCN

On September 10, 2001, I headed to Washington, District of Columbia, aboard Amtrak. After working the day at the hospital, I headed to the nation's capitol to spend three days reviewing grants for the United States Department of Education. The trip seemed as though it would be a learning, skill-building and networking experience. Before departing the hospital, as was my habit, I left phone numbers for the hotel and my cell phone and an e-mail address where I could be reached while away.

The morning of September 11, I was in an orientation meeting, when a representative from the hotel came in to interrupt the meeting with an announcement. She informed us that two planes had gone into the World Trade Center, and she said there was speculation that a third plane had gone into the Department of Treasury building in lower Manhattan. (At this time, we did not know about the downed planes at the Pentagon or in Pennsylvania). She told us this was considered to be an act of war, not an accident. We were also informed that all of our cell phones were down and that regular phone service was sporadic. As if we could not process the lost communication information, nearly every person in the room attempted to use their cell phone instantaneously. No one got through.

I recall the meeting leader informing us that this was most likely an act of terrorists. He further stated that terrorists seek to disrupt business and cause chaos. We were told we had two choices, since we could not travel because of the citywide lock-down. We could: (1) return to our

[Haworth co-indexing entry note]: "Personal Perspective on 9/11." Burkhardt, Ann. Co-published simultaneously in *Occupational Therapy in Mental Health* (The Haworth Press, Inc.) Vol. 19, No. 3/4, 2003, pp. 59-71; and: *Surviving 9/11: Impact and Experiences of Occupational Therapy Practitioners* (ed: Pat Precin) The Haworth Press, Inc., 2003, pp. 59-71. Single or multiple copies of this article are available for a fee from The Haworth Document Delivery Service [1-800-HAWORTH, 9:00 a.m. - 5:00 p.m. (EST). E-mail address: docdelivery@haworthpress.com].

Digital Object Identifier: 10.1300/J004v19n03_06

rooms and be overwhelmed by the circumstances; or (2) adjourn for two hours to contact our families any way we were able and then carry on with the business we had come to do. As we were all attempting to gather our thoughts and to have a moment of clarity, the hotel representative again entered the room to announce that a third plane had gone into the Pentagon. At that moment, I knew I would need to contact my parents in Rhode Island and my brother in New York State. No one had a clear idea of where I was in Washington. I knew I was not near the Pentagon, but I was ignorant as to my location, just six blocks from the White House (which I had not realized was a potential target).

I returned to my hotel room and dialed Rhode Island. My folks were out, but their answering machine picked up. "I am all right," I said. "The Pentagon is at the other end of Washington. I am staying put for the time being. It seems it is probably safer just to stay put for now. The cell phones are down, but I will try to call back again later." Then I dialed my brother's home in Rochester, New York. My sister-in-law answered. She filled me in on additional details of what had occurred. She agreed to share news of my well-being with our family.

My work group convened to discuss our plan for the day. We made a pact to review our grants and to occasionally get updates from the television. The five of us had six grants to review. We received our assigned grants and broke for lunch. One of the people in the group had extensive experience with this process. He agreed to begin the review that afternoon. We stuck to task and supported each other as time progressed.

During a break, I successfully phoned an occupational therapy colleague in Virginia whose husband had been recently assigned to the Pentagon. She reported that he had an appointment outside of the building that day, so thankfully was not in danger (L. Comis, personal communication, September 11, 2001). A native New Yorker, she reported she had been unable to reach anyone in New York since the accident.

My initial reaction was to feel as though I had "abandoned ship." Here I was several hundred miles away from New York. My staff in New York City was unreachable by phone. News reports stated that the hospitals were on high alert, prepared for disaster throughout the city. The initial speculation was that there would be many people, some burned, that would have to be triaged to hospitals throughout the Tri-state area. Having been through disaster drills at my facility, I visualized what the staff and facility must be doing and the internal atmosphere. The summer before, the staff had had practice. Our facility was hit with a blackout. All of the power had gone down and everyone assumed new duties and roles–from running ice up six floors, to fanning patients in hot, non-air-conditioned intensive care units to manually pumping air for people who were dependent on respirators.

That afternoon I e-mailed several staff members. Initially I thought that the e-mail system might also be down. Surprisingly, I got a return response (and actually found an e-mail message awaiting me when I logged into the system). The staff was on high alert. Regular therapy treatment had been interrupted. There had been an hourly administrative update. One supervisor attended and circulated updates to the staff. They were informed that they might be needed into the evening. However, by the late afternoon, no survivors were arriving at area emergency rooms north of 96th street in Manhattan. It was becoming clear that hospitals were probably not going to be receiving large numbers of wounded survivors. As the day progressed, we began to actualize the probable number of deaths from the attack.

Some members of our staff were recalling a vivid visual image. When the planes were approaching the World Trade Center, they flew at a low altitude down the Hudson River–just above the parapets of the George Washington Bridge. The physical therapy gym on our rehabilitation unit looks out at the bridge and the river. When the aides in our department saw the planes, they ran around to the opposite side of the building. From the sky bridges, they watched the planes hit the towers. The skyways at our facility have a clear view straight down the length of Manhattan. The stories have since been repeated and repeated with clarity of detail and continuing disbelief that this occurred here in New York City.

Outside of my hotel, I stood momentarily in disbelief, as I watched lines of traffic evacuating the downtown area. They were all leaving town, but we could not. Those of us who were housed in hotels were comfortable to a degree, but sick at heart over the events and our isolation. I was reminded of a scene from a film, where everyone evacuates a city after a nuclear bomb has been dropped. Would we all survive this? I became aware of the sound of military planes flying overhead. I saw military vehicles driving along the streets. This was a New World that had emerged seemingly overnight.

By evening, given the "green light" from hospital administration, most of the staff began to formulate and execute plans for getting home to their families. All of the bridge crossings were closed. Buses and subways did not run. Some of the therapists who lived close by in Manhattan offered a place to sleep to colleagues. A group of the staff from the Bronx started out on foot, walked to and crossed one of the bridges. A family member met them on the opposite side. The pediatric therapists opted to bed down in the clinic on mats–forming makeshift sleeping quarters with blankets and pillows, washing up in the sink and "roughing it." The therapists from New Jersey, who drive daily across the George Washington Bridge, began to contemplate what it would be like for them in the future driving across the bridge. The news reported that the bridge was on the list of potential targets. Any sense of feeling safe or secure on one's ride to work was eliminated.

Another alliance was forged that day in New Jersey. The mothers of two acute care therapists who commute across the bridge phoned each other to discuss the probable status of their daughters. They could not telephone Manhattan. They could only speculate that the girls were all right. Meanwhile therapists were dreading their next passage across the bridge. In reality, they were safe, but suffering from the events of the day and the media speculation that more planes or bombs could be coming. As weeks passed, one therapist began supportive therapy for a developing phobia of crossing the bridge. The other admitted her trepidation as well, but opted to work through her fears by "getting back on the horse."

At 7:30 p.m., I was mesmerized in front of the television set in my hotel room. Saddened and in disbelief, I was feeling lost and guilty for being away from New York at a time when I speculated that my skills in burns and acute care could be best used. My cell phone rang. One colleague, with whom I had worked for twenty-two years, phoned from her home in the Bronx. She had reached home safely and wanted to know if I was safe. After our conversation, another friend and colleague phoned my cell phone to ask about my whereabouts and safety. They both reassured me that all was well. They had been inconvenienced, but everyone was all right. Several members of the department, whose husbands or other family members worked downtown, were fine. One staff member's cousin had a fiancée who was missing. That was all the anticipated personal losses amongst my staff. This was amazing and positive news.

By the second day, lines of communication opened with friends and family. My family was concerned, but feeling supported by the outpouring of phone calls and messages from family and friends around the world and the nation. They were concerned about my eventual need to travel, but continued to support the decision to stay in Washington until the train began moving again, and I could travel back to New York City.

My Dad suffers occasionally with Post-Traumatic Stress Syndrome related to his front line experiences in the Pacific during World War II. Both he and my Mom related what was happening back to war years–especially where they were and what happened on Pearl Harbor

Day. They both reassured me that we would get back to some sense of normalcy once again, but that it would take time and effort to bring about change.

Throughout my stay, I was in close contact with a close colleague in Manhattan. She is a native New Yorker. She spoke with my folks, concerned about my whereabouts. This colleague also shared her perceptions of what was happening in her neighborhood, near Lincoln Center on the Upper West Side of Manhattan (K. Stone, personal communication, September 21, 2001) (see Appendix). Signs of patriotism emerged. People stopped and shared thoughts and experiences with neighbors. Families and friends went out of their way to communicate. Through her eyes, I began to sense community in the midst of profound sadness. We cried together on the phone as she told me of the small girl in the building who taped a hand-drawn American flag to the front door.

In addition to the people who are generally tangible in my life, I had begun an online doctoral program only one month before September 11th. I now had a connection to a larger community of occupational therapists on-line. My virtual campus was centered in Omaha, Nebraska. The President of the United States was whisked off to Omaha early in the day of September 11th, because of its strategic military location. Some of the people who had been aboard the flight in Pennsylvania were also from Omaha. The impact of the disaster had reached beyond New York and Washington. I became aware that the losses from all of the attacks had touched people across the nation. Our assignment that week was postponed. We chatted on-line with each other. We learned of family and friends of classmates who had been touched by the events. I spoke with one classmate several times by phone from my hotel room that week.

By Friday, September 14, I was on my way back to Pennsylvania Station, New York. Upon reaching the station and the street, I was pleased to find taxicabs and public transportation running. As I headed up to my neighborhood on the Upper East Side, the sight of armed military walking the streets awed me (Photo 1). At the 68th Street Armory, there were humvees lining the street outside. The ordinarily pristine Park Avenue was unevenly adorned with American flags of all sizes and quality. Large flags draped over the fronts of buildings (Photo 2).

Upon reaching home, I learned that a woman in my apartment building was unaccounted for. The neighbors were unclear whether she was traveling or missing. That evening and for several evenings following it, there were candlelight vigils (Photo 3).

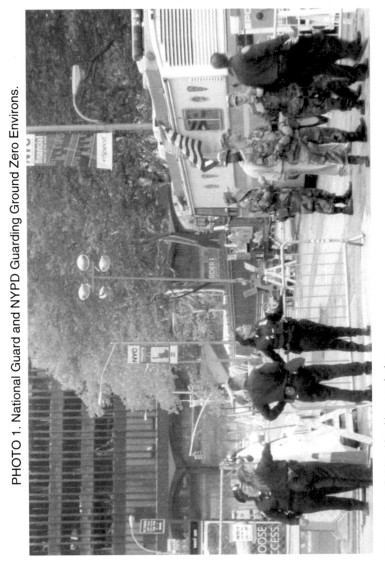

PHOTO 1. National Guard and NYPD Guarding Ground Zero Environs.

Photo by Fran Babiss. Used by permission.

PHOTO 2. Large Flag Hanging from a Ground Zero Building. The Dedication Below Reads, "Thank You For Not Giving Up. We Will Never Forget Them. We Will Never Forget You. Love, The WTC Families. We Love NY."

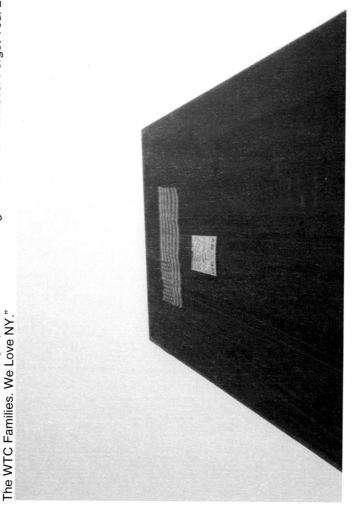

Photo by Pat Precin. Used by permission.

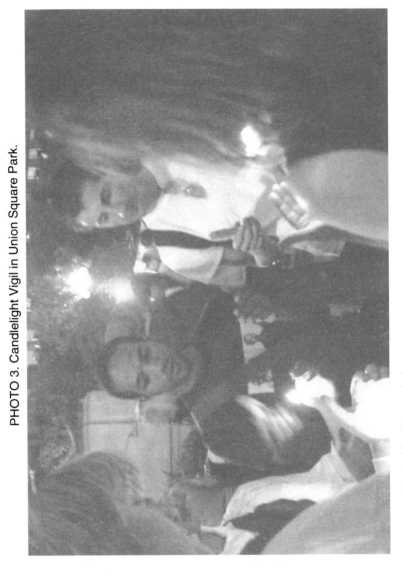

PHOTO 3. Candlelight Vigil in Union Square Park.

Photo by Pat Precin. Used by permission.

By the second week, many of the occupational therapists in my department and near my community were discussing (live and on-line) their desire to volunteer at Ground Zero. When we contacted the Red Cross, we were told that we were not included in their list of qualified mental health providers. Our help was not wanted. Also, when some of us who have training in massage techniques offered to assist with caring for workers at Ground Zero, we were told they would only consider using massage and physical therapists. Only one person from my staff, an attractive advanced clinical pediatric occupational therapist, was accepted to work the worker relief unit (Johansson, 2002). She went to Ground Zero with physical therapy colleagues who fought for her inclusion. She was issued identification and allowed to help.

I brought this to the attention of the national leadership of the profession, who were surprised to hear of this situation, since the occupational therapists in the military were those who were doing most of the debriefing from the Pentagon (Gourley, 2002). However, we agreed that the military has consistently offered Critical Incident Stress Debriefing training to occupational therapists, and this was not offered to non-military professionals. We lacked the strategic training that had made our colleagues sought after as primary interventionists.

Within that week, I heard reports from colleagues at Mount Sinai Hospital that they had decided to go directly to the firehouses in their vicinity and offer direct help (R. Sable, personal communication, 2001). Their offer had been welcomed and their services accepted. We heard stories of their transportation back to their neighborhoods via fire engine, after connecting with tired emergency workers who were grateful for their therapy services.

The following weeks also led to opportunities for occupational therapists in White Plains. The Red Cross had accepted them to assist with interviewing and processing reports from families with missing relatives from the World Trade Center. Several therapists did assist in White Plains.

In November, New York held its state conference in Albany. A colleague, who rode to Albany with me, told a story of a friend, an artist in the World Trade Center, who was killed on 9/11. Michael Richards' (1963-2001) art had focused on the Tuskeegee Airmen (Richards, 2002). One statue in particular pictured planes flying into a larger-than-life size by comparison airman. My colleague stated how uncanny this work had been. Michael's studio was at the probable point of impact of the first plane. His art seemed prophetic, karmic. My colleague shared that her family and friends had some sense of relief, because parts of his body were found and identified. They knew he was dead. My colleague reported that they all experienced profound loss, but at least had had closure about their friend.

During the annual state conference in Albany, our New York State Occupational Therapy President, Sue Seiler, shared an outpouring of support and financial assistance that had come to us from our colleagues in California. At their annual conference, just following 9/11, they circulated paper for personal messages and took up a collection. The messages warmed our hearts, left us in tears and gave us a sense of hope and connection with our colleagues from the opposite coast. President Seiler challenged us to contribute equally and to found a fund to assist occupational therapy colleagues who could not afford to participate in our community in the aftereffect of the attack. A collection was taken and a fund was set up.

We also learned that the American Occupational Therapy Association President, Barbara Kornblau, herself a New Yorker by birth, had lost a young cousin in the World Trade Center. Her cousin had recently married. She reported to work on the morning of 9/11 and was presumed dead. Months later, during the Annual American Occupational Therapy Association Conference in Miami in May 2002, colleagues presented Barbara with a special patriotic card. Inside were personal messages and a photograph of her with her cousin. As I faced the podium at which members of the American Occupational Therapy Association Executive Board sat, there were many tears shed. This single act brought us together as a national group. It forced our remembrance of September 11th of the past year. No matter how far away from September 11th in time or distance, the profound sadness prevailed and would prevail in our hearts throughout our lifetimes.

August arrives in New York this week. The record player in my head wants to play my favorite autumn song about New York. My mind remembers the fond, romantic tune, but my heart knows that this autumn will bring back tears and remembrance of things we will never forget. Our generation has experienced its Pearl Harbor. We have been changed forever. We have been strengthened. Our sleep is still erratic. Irrational fears could be rational, depending on circumstance. Change beyond our control occurred. We are alive but vigilant.

September 11, 2002 will be here soon. We all live in hope that America will stand united in our loss. We also live in hope that we will sense renewed security and freedom once again. In reflection, how have the events changed our lives, our patterns, and our occupations? How are we coping with the events of the past year?

I personally feel that we take each other less for granted. Over the past year, I have made an effort to connect and reconnect with friends and colleagues who have also reached out to me. It seems to me that we are all more patient and less concerned about cooperating with security measures. People share stories of how they were searched or planes were delayed, but generally, there is complacency with delays. There is a shared renewed value in feeling safe and secure. If security does not live up to its purported stringency, there is alarm. It appears appreciated that we would rather "be safe than sorry."

There also seems to be renewed patriotism. A few years ago, signs of patriotism were scoffed at. Now, red, white and blue clothing is at a premium. Everyone seems to applaud the military and veterans, in general.

Perhaps one aspect of daily life that has been most disrupted, and about which I continuously seem to hear people speak, is sleep. Lack of sleep, disturbed sleep, altered sleep habits, and nightmares all are fair fodder for conversation. I find myself believing that it is a normal reaction after the enormity of terror we all collectively experienced. Is it odd to worry about our degree of prevalence of Post-Traumatic Stress Disorder? I find myself questioning whether it is truly a disorder at all, if most of the population is experiencing it.

Currently, I am in the midst of doing community-based well-elderly research. Many of the people I meet in Northern Manhattan share what they were doing on September 11. Part of the study involves an anxiety and depression index. The evidence has to be compiled before conclusions can be drawn, but as a casual observer, many of those I meet who are over 65 seem least affected by post-9/11 stress. Many of them lived through World War II. September 11th was sad and unfortunate, but survivors value the process and participation in living.

I worry the most about the spouses of friends and colleagues who lost lifelong friends and family members in the disaster. Their lives have experienced the greatest loss and I am unsure how "friends" have been treated in the recovery from the disaster. Some friendships are closer than marriages. I personally wish someone would measure the levels of depression and anxiety amongst those who lost peers. We have had our attention drawn to firefighters and police officers and their loss, but no one has paid due homage to the businessperson who once worked in the World Trade Center and who lost his childhood friend at Cantor Fitzgerald.

It seems to me that resources, such as the services of Project Liberty (2002), exist, but are under-utilized by New Yorkers who want to get on with life, but who still experience a twinge each time a state of heightened alert is announced, or the governor increases troops in Pennsylvania Station.

As a manager, I have not noticed increased use of sick time, or abuses of time as one might suspect when people are under stress. There does seem to be a heightened willingness to cooperate and accommodate each other when staff members need time for family or personal matters. Members of our department have had two babies this year and two more babies are due within the next six months. I perceive that we are being more humanistic, more willing to "give an inch," more willing to "go the extra mile," but also very interested in living our lives more fully than we have since the computer age emerged.

Anniversaries can be prophetic. We will wait, listen, learn, and live through the ones to come. September 11, 2002 will be the first of many.

REFERENCES

Comis, L. (2001). Personal communication, September 11.

Gourley, M. (2002). *OTs on the front lines.* Retrieved August 15, 2002, from *http://www.aota.org/nonmembers/area1/links/link222.asp*

Johansson, C. (2002). *Occupational therapy helps heal a nation.* Retrieved August 15, 2002, from *http://www.aota.org/nonmembers/area1/links/link209.asp*

Project Liberty. (n.d.). Retrieved August 15, 2002, from *www.projectliberty.state.ny.us*

Richards, M. (2002). The power of flight. *New York University Steinhardt School of Education Alumni News, 13*(2), pp. 1 & 5.

APPENDIX
Letter to Betty [Ann] and Ken Burkhardt

Karen L. Stone, MA,OTR/L
24 West 69th Street 9A
New York, NY 10023
(212) 362-4551

September 21, 2002

Dear Betty and Ken [Burkhardt],

I write to thank you for your phone calls and messages. Your expressions of concern were so important to us. Those first days we felt so isolated from the rest of the United States and the world. We didn't know how others felt about us and if they felt like Jerry Falwell later expressed he felt. We didn't know if others understood the horror we were experiencing.

On Tuesday, 9/11/01, I could not bring myself to unchain my front door. The phones didn't work at first, and when they did we couldn't make long distance calls. Everyone locally was trying to find out if everyone they knew was still alive. The sounds were those of sirens blaring and fighter jets flying back and forth overhead. I looked out of the window with the view of Central Park West and saw steady throngs of people walking north. There was no transportation and people were walking home wherever that was or walking away. It was hard to sleep that night.

On Wednesday, 9/12/01, I left my home. The streets were silent except when people met and asked each other whether they and theirs were okay. By then, we knew no one in the United States was safe anymore. The other sound was of F-16 fighter jets patrolling the air space over New York City. I went to a Memorial Service that night. Most of us just couldn't be comforted. Afterwards outside, the winds had changed and the smell of smoke was very strong.

On Thursday, 9/13/01, I walked across Central Park to Gloria's (my daughter) house to take her out to lunch. Because of Louis, 2½, they were trying to keep the horror out of their home. She needed to be free to talk and cry. The city was never so filled with sound. The trucks, the taxis, the people on their cell phones, it was as if everything and everyone was shouting, "I am alive! I survived!"

The initial shock and horror were swiftly followed by numbness, which is giving way to pain, fear and anger. People complain of being very tired, of feeling overwhelmed and unable to focus on things. It is so easy to cry and it feels so good to do so. We are developing new skills. I can now realize the sound of a fighter jet and distinguish it from a passenger jet. Which way the wind is blowing matters because the smell of smoke is so pungent. Sadness is very visible too. I see it on other faces and I feel its heaviness on me.

The funerals have begun for those few who have a body. The memorial services for the multitude without a body have begun too. The newspaper obituaries are filled with those lost on 9/11/01 and many, many of them are in their 30's. Our local firehouse lost 11.

We all seem suspended in time and disbelief while at the same time waiting for the next attack. But we are very united as Americans in this melting pot of a city where every nationality, color, religion, and sexual and political choice has its origin on its American journey. We have been reduced to an equality and oneness of purpose that would make our founding fathers very proud. We are where America begins. Perhaps that is why it was so important for the terrorists to destroy us.

Thank you for calling. Thank you for letting them share of my sorrow with you. Please know that along with such pain our city is filled with courage, faith, and hope. We know that love is stronger than hate. The sleeping cat is awake and it is a tiger and it is fierce and it is us. Thanks again,

Karen

September Twelfth:
An American Away from Home

Jennifer Wright, MS, OTR, NZROT

I woke up as usual, making my way sleepy-eyed to my computer, which sat in my living room. The sun had not yet peeked over the eastern horizon, which I could see out of my wonderful big window. My house sits high above the city and I could see the city lights dancing away in the distance. This morning ritual of reading my e-mails is performed for two reasons. First, living halfway round the world, in New Zealand, I wake up to messages from friends from the United States who are already up and about while I, a day later, am stumbling out of bed. Second, the man in my life, Aad, lives seven hours away from me, so we communicate via Internet Messenger every morning when we are each at our respective homes.

I opened my first e-mail that morning to a puzzling message from a dear friend, Arlis, entitled *Terrible Thing*. It read, "I am sure you have seen the news; I hope they find the bastards who did this," but nothing more. I was stunned. What was he talking about? As I wondered, I saw the little green figure light up signaling that Aad was logging on to Messenger in order to communicate with me. He wrote, "Someone has bombed the Pentagon."

I quickly turned on the television and heard the American Broadcasting Company news being broadcast with American accents. With the television at my back, I picked up flashes of a story while I wrote back

[Haworth co-indexing entry note]: "September Twelfth: An American Away from Home." Wright, Jennifer. Co-published simultaneously in *Occupational Therapy in Mental Health* (The Haworth Press, Inc.) Vol. 19, No. 3/4, 2003, pp. 73-77; and: *Surviving 9/11: Impact and Experiences of Occupational Therapy Practitioners* (ed: Pat Precin) The Haworth Press, Inc., 2003, pp. 73-77. Single or multiple copies of this article are available for a fee from The Haworth Document Delivery Service [1-800-HAWORTH, 9:00 a.m. - 5:00 p.m. (EST). E-mail address: docdelivery@haworthpress.com].

and forth to Aad, trying to piece things together. My first thought was, *Oh my God, another Tim McVey,* then I thought, *What tortured soul would do this?* I was having such a hard time understanding what had happened. The television showed pictures of smoke, fire and flashes of people screaming and running. New York City's Twin Towers! I thought, *How could this be happening to my beloved America?* By this time, I realized this was not the act of a disgruntled American. This was a terrorist attack! I signed off with Aad and we promised each other to try to figure out what had happened.

I was becoming sick and felt like I was in a daze. I wanted to throw up, cry, and scream. I live on my own and felt very alone. I called my parents. They did not answer. However, the sound of their voice on the answering machine was music to my ears, and I told them so. My adult children I knew would be working or at school.

I began to get myself ready for work. I work as a lecturer at Otago Polytechnic School of Occupational Therapy in Dunedin. The 12th of September started our weeks of final examinations. Students are examined orally. Students are given a case study and asked to identify and defend a plan of intervention, state which frames of reference they used and cite literature. I had to face a day of orally examining eight students. I needed to stop pacing around the house and focus my efforts on getting to work.

I walked to work (30 minutes) crying on and off. I wanted to talk to someone about what was happening. When I arrived at work, a staff member who expressed shock at what was happening in the United States immediately approached me. Before I could respond another staff member said, "Americans! They bomb the hell out of everyone else on the planet and then wonder why they get bombed!"

I could not say anything. I was stunned. Fortunately, the rest of the staff and students treated me quite kindly. I was asked if I thought that I could actually give the oral examinations. I said, "Yes," knowing that delays would mean delays for students going on fieldwork placements. I was asked many times, "Do you have family in New York?" Of course I said, "No, I am from Indiana." What I felt like saying was, *This is my country that has been attacked, it is my home! It is bigger than having family in New York!*

I had much trouble concentrating on the exams. My mind would drift back to thoughts of people, people who went to work that day just like me and did not come home. I felt disconnected and guilty that I was not in the United States. Selfish me–I had left for this adventure around the world and was not connected to this event. I would try very hard to connect to the students I was examining, trying hard not to let my thoughts drift. Sometimes, I could not control the drifting and I would find myself trying, again, to figure out what had happened. As a result, I would have to ask the students to repeat themselves. *Sometimes, I told myself, there is nothing I could do at this moment for anyone but pray.* I prayed so many times: *Lord whatever part I have had in this hatred that created this atrocity, please forgive me.*

I believed that I, through my own thoughts of hatred, could be a part of this destructive act. I needed to connect somehow. Throughout the day, people stopped me, expressing their concern, recognizing me as an American. I still felt numb. I went to a prayer vigil that night in the center of town. I felt very disconnected and alone. That night I went home and watched the news again and tried to understand. I missed being *there.* I wanted desperately to know what my old friends and neighbors were saying, not what the American Broadcasting Company news was telecasting. What did my American friends think was happening? But it was too late to call anyone.

Not long after arriving home that evening, a call came from my friend Hans, who works for the Otago *Daily Times,* the regional newspaper. He told me he was bringing me a copy of the special edition newspaper. When he arrived a few minutes later, I was unprepared for "Civilization Under Terrorist Attack" as headlines and a full-page picture of the burning Twin Towers. I wondered if this could really be happening in my homeland.

As the week wore on, I continued to communicate with friends via e-mail. Many messages included pictures of the heroism of the American people. I felt so proud and wanted to reach out to someone. I felt that no one in New Zealand really understood what it is like to be an American at this time of tragedy, being heroic, being proud in the way that we are. I got my American flag out and, having no place to hang it outside, hung it inside.

I watched the news and read commentaries and tried so very hard to understand the desperation involved in people that would do such a thing. I also thought of other world events, people dying and getting much less media attention. I asked myself, *Why should there be a difference in degree of importance between an American death due to this tragedy and someone else's death?*

The New Zealand press is very pro-American, as are most of the New Zealand people. Their reactions to the disaster were mostly sympathetic and publicly expressed through newspapers, radio broadcasts, television, public gatherings, prayer services and memorial services. However, these reports were lacking the depth and analysis that American media was portraying. I missed the "experts" discussing at lengths different ways of looking at the situation to help me understand beyond the news story. Many people expressed concern and fear of a World War III.

I received many calls from friends and acquaintances (New Zealanders) during the first week after the twelfth of September. People were very generous with their gifts showing sympathy and concern for me. Students were also concerned about my well-being and that of my family. Many poked their heads into my office and told me so.

I wrote two letters to people I felt I needed to ask for forgiveness from events in my past. I felt that my unresolved issues added negativity to the universal energy that helped create this disaster. This was how I made sense of my connection and responsibility for this situation.

Aad arrived the weekend after the disaster and we talked through our fears. I had planned a year ago to fly home for a visit on September 20th. We felt afraid about my flying back to Indiana. Many people expressed opinions about how crazy I was to fly to the States now. I heard warnings from both sides of the Pacific: "How can you do such a dangerous thing?" Aad and I sat and cried and held each other contemplating this flight. He wanted to go with me, but we could not afford such a trip. We had a sense of dread, yet I knew that I would go if I was allowed. I just needed to physically touch base with home. I needed to see Americans.

Both my children, especially my son, expressed concern about my flying at this time. I explained to him quite honestly that I was willing to take my chances. I needed to touch base for many reasons and there were things worse than dying. One of those was living in fear.

I arrived home on the 20th of September. I will never forget the American flags at an empty Los Angeles International Airport. This airport is usually so busy that you need to be aggressive to make your way through the crowds to make a connecting flight. I will always remember the heartwarming patriotic music playing in the desolate Chicago O'Hare Airport and the Los Angeles customs' agent saying, "Welcome home, Jennifer!"

I spent nearly three weeks with my family and friends. I was overwhelmed by the patriotism: flags on cars, T-shirts and lapel pins. I was able to experience what I had longed for, the average American's dealing with this tragedy. I listened to talk radio, attended church, spoke and debated with friends and family, and listened to news commentaries. I watched several popular politically incorrect television shows that utilized satire and comedy to bring different perspectives of the disaster to public awareness. I watched a sad show that replayed people's final calls home during the disaster. I drove my friend's pickup truck and listened to country western music because they played so many patriotic songs. I could not access country western music in New Zealand. I found people in New York to be friendly and helpful, as if something inside them was awakened by this unthinkable event. I think they found happiness in waking up everyday, performing their occupations with gratitude, and treating each other with respect. They were optimistic and determined.

I wanted to absorb as much as I could to "take back with me" to New Zealand, my adopted home. I brought country western music, a pair of blue jeans, a cowboy hat, and a "Proud to be an American" pin that I sometimes rub my hands across and remember. I brought back the hope that this tragedy will not be forgotten and that people will remember the joy of living and the blessing of forgiveness.

Ground Zero Needs Assessment

Pat Precin, MS, OTR/L

Frank R. Pascarelli, Occupational Therapist, Biomedical Science Corps Officer and Former Firefighter, returned to his hometown, New York City, when called to duty by the United States Air Force on September 11th to conduct a needs assessment at Ground Zero. The following is a description of his findings.

* * *

As I traveled to Ground Zero, the security progressively tightened as I came closer to the site of the fallen towers. I can still remember as I walked from my car to the plaza of the World Trade Center how very quiet it was, except for the sounds of heavy equipment removing the debris (Photos 1-7). The rubble piles were still smoldering and the air was heavy and gritty (Photos 8-10).

When I began to work with the [recovery] crews, I noticed certain signs of stress among the workers: speaking in a monotone or not speaking

[Haworth co-indexing entry note]: "Ground Zero Needs Assessment." Precin, Pat. Co-published simultaneously in *Occupational Therapy in Mental Health* (The Haworth Press, Inc.) Vol. 19, No. 3/4, 2003, pp. 79-101; and: *Surviving 9/11: Impact and Experiences of Occupational Therapy Practitioners* (ed: Pat Precin) The Haworth Press, Inc., 2003, pp. 79-101. Single or multiple copies of this article are available for a fee from The Haworth Document Delivery Service [1-800-HAWORTH, 9:00 a.m. - 5:00 p.m. (EST). E-mail address: docdelivery@haworthpress.com].

Digital Object Identifier: 10.1300/J004v19n03_08

PHOTO 1. Heavy Equipment Moving Debris.

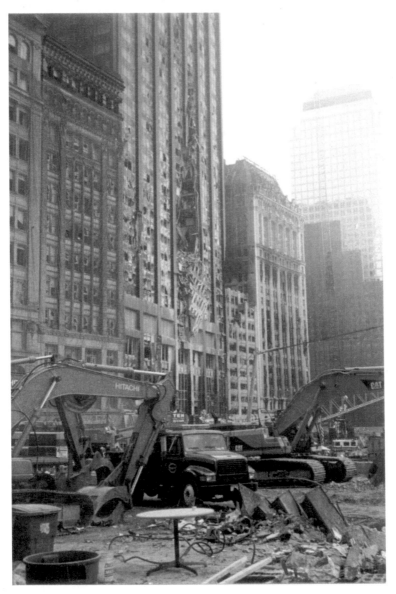

Photo by Frank Pascarelli. Used by permission.

PHOTO 2. Heavy Equipment Moving Debris.

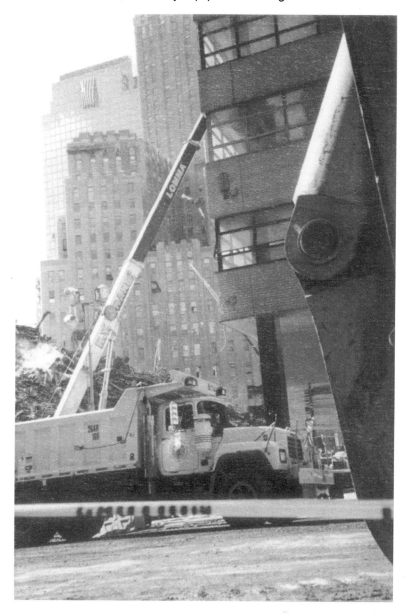

Photo by Frank Pascarelli. Used by permission.

PHOTO 3. Ground Zero

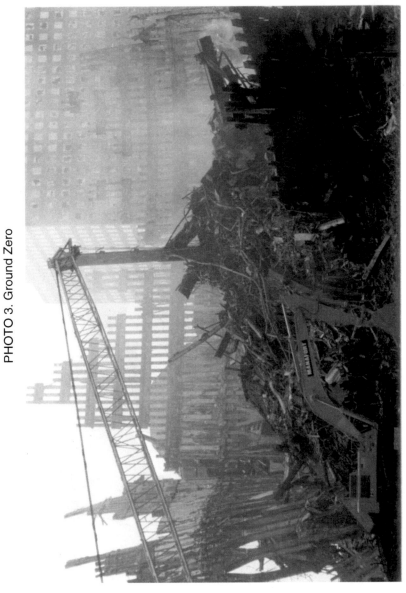

Photo by Frank Pascarelli. Used by permission.

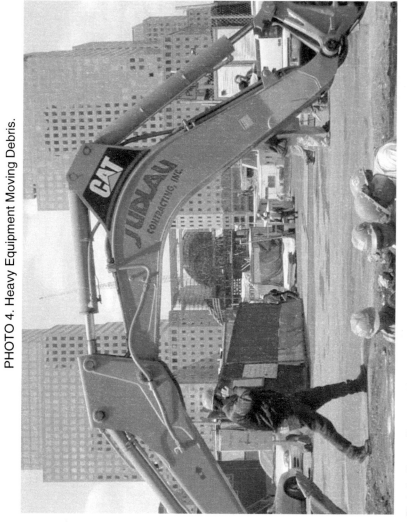

PHOTO 4. Heavy Equipment Moving Debris.

Photo by Donna Brennan. Used by permission.

PHOTO 5. Working Around the Clock

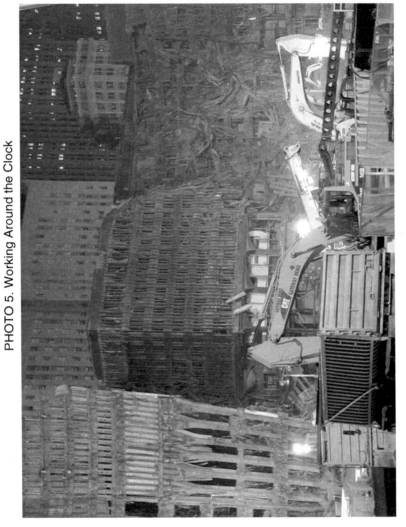

Photo by Donna Brennan. Used by permission.

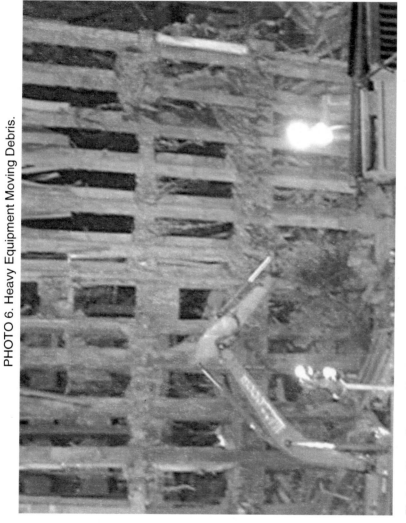

PHOTO 6. Heavy Equipment Moving Debris.

Photo by Donna Brennan. Used by permission.

PHOTO 7. Onlooker.

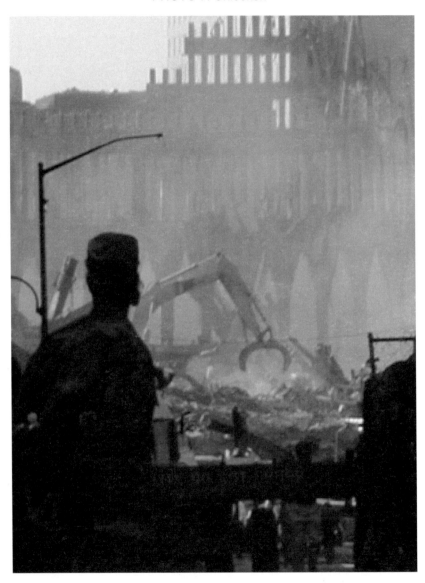

Photo by Donna Brennan. Used by permission.

PHOTO 8. Workers Wearing Masks as Ground Zero Continues to Smolder.

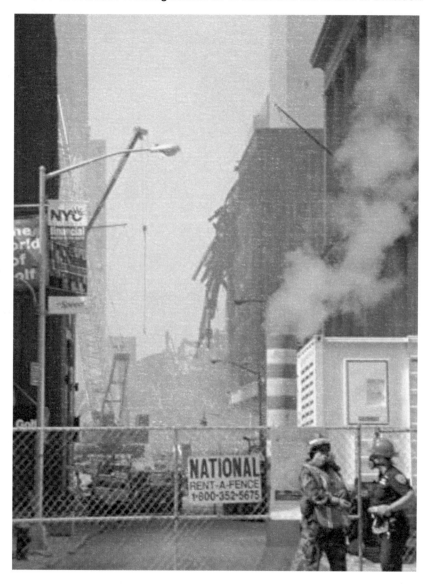

Photo by Donna Brennan. Used by permission.

PHOTO 9. Ground Zero at Night.

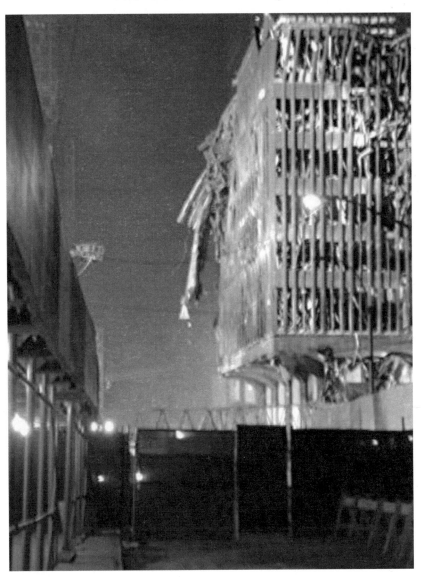

Photo by Donna Brennan. Used by permission.

PHOTO 10. Massive Destruction

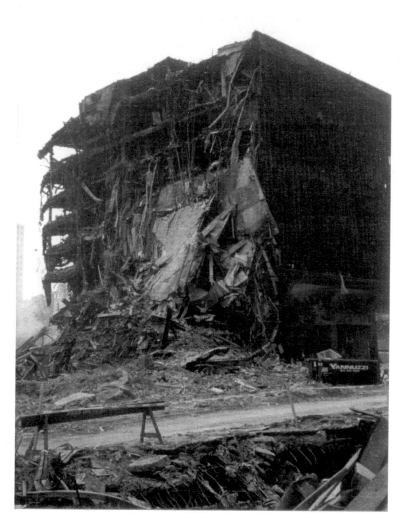

Photo by Frank Pascarelli. Used by permission.

at all, having no facial expression, moving deliberately, avoiding eye contact, and withdrawing from others (Photos 11-12). (These behaviors may be an attempt to overcome, escape or adapt to stress.) Environmental stressors at Ground Zero included: noise, extremes in temperature, fumes that include irritants, obscure vision from small particles of dust and large dust clouds, confined work spaces, and an unstable (and unsafe) work environment (Photo 13). Physiological stressors included: sleep deprivation, dehydration, injury, fatigue and poor hygiene. Emotional stressors (Photo 14) included: fear, anxiety, grief, anger, frustration, resentment, guilt, and spiritual conflict. Cognitive stressors included sensory overload, information overload, and unpredictability.

PHOTO 11. Recovery Crew with Hardhats, Eye Shields, and Masks.

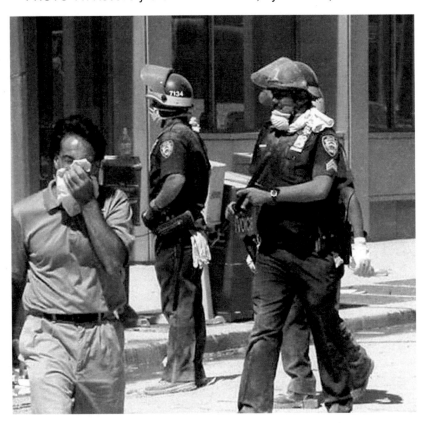

Photo by Gilad Rosner. Used by permission.

PHOTO 12. Recovery Crew.

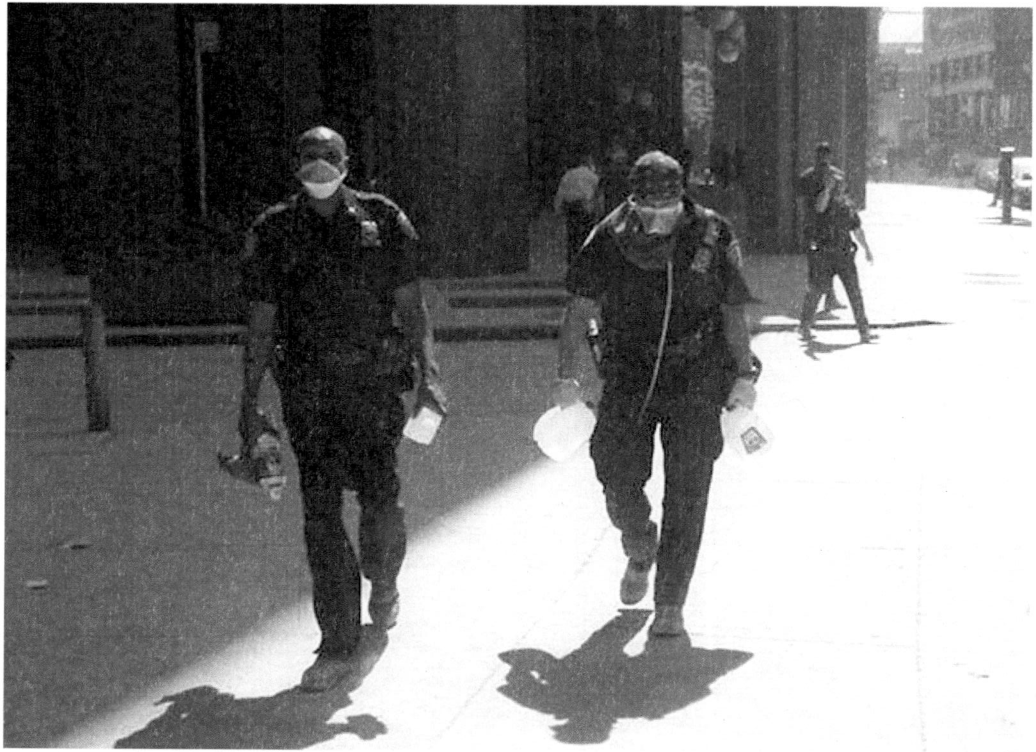

Photo by Gilad Rosner. Used by permission.

91

PHOTO 13. Working in Isolation with Irritant Fumes and Obscured Vision in an Unstable Environment Are Environmental Stressors Experienced at Ground Zero.

92

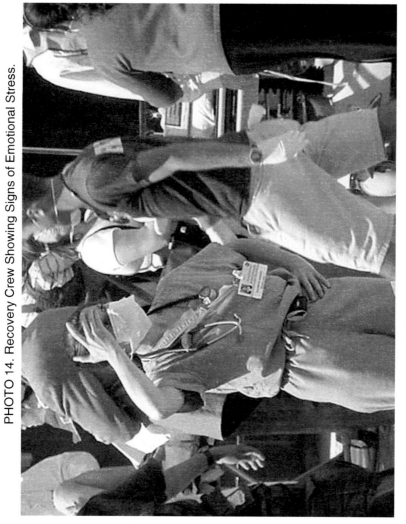

PHOTO 14. Recovery Crew Showing Signs of Emotional Stress.

Photo by Gilad Rosner. Used by permission.

These individuals had gone well beyond the point of exhaustion. Many had not left the site since the attacks. They ate and slept inside the "zone" (Photo 15). Several supervisors told me some of the workers had forgotten the world outside the fence. Groups stayed together and did everything together at the same time. Some workers had reservations about their ability to return to their jobs when this was all over. Other workers were not concerned about their own safety, just the safety of the victims and that of the "city." There is an understanding in the fire service; you do not leave a scene without all your men. As a former firefighter, I understood this, but as an occupational therapist, I was concerned about the firefighters' ability to reintegrate into their previous roles after the site closed.

Many of the workers I came into contact with at Ground Zero welcomed an opportunity to express their feelings as long as they could still work at the same time. Since it was difficult to do both, the firefighters harbored many unresolved issues. Many firefighters were working around the clock. Relief crews and supervisors recognized the need for a balance of work, self-care and rest, but the challenge was getting the firefighters to do it. Showers and tents were brought in to allow the teams to address their activities of daily living needs (Photo 16), and clothing exchange points were set up. Workers could wash their masks at various "mask washing stations" (Photo 17).

As time went on, there was mounting anxiety amongst the firefighters regarding how long the operation would be classified as "rescue" before it became a "recovery" mission. They wanted to continue to search for live bodies as long as possible. They were dreading the day when officials would decrease the number of firefighters at the site. I thought the change from rescue to recovery presented the biggest challenge for the officials in charge of the operation because it signified that there would be little if any chance of finding someone alive. The second problem was how to scale back the crews at the site. Who was going to decide who could stay and dig and for how long and who was going to leave? The longer these two issues took to implement, the harder it was going to be to make the transition. On the other hand, the American people were not ready for the transition. They wanted to believe there was some chance, some glimmer of hope among all the destruction that somehow, somewhere there could be someone alive. This affected the timing of the decision and fueled the dedication of the rescuers (Photos 18-19).

* * *

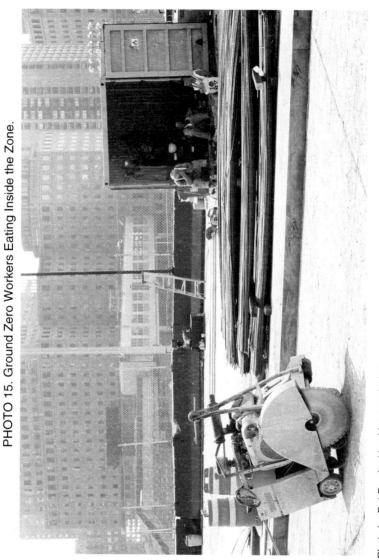

PHOTO 15. Ground Zero Workers Eating Inside the Zone.

Photo by Pat Precin. Used by permission.

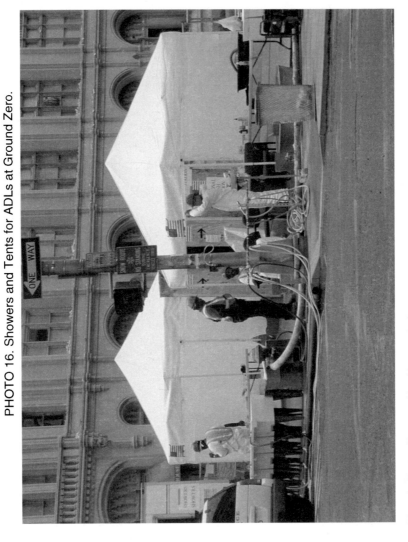

PHOTO 16. Showers and Tents for ADLs at Ground Zero.

Photo by Donna Brennan. Used by permission.

PHOTO 17. Mask Washing Station.

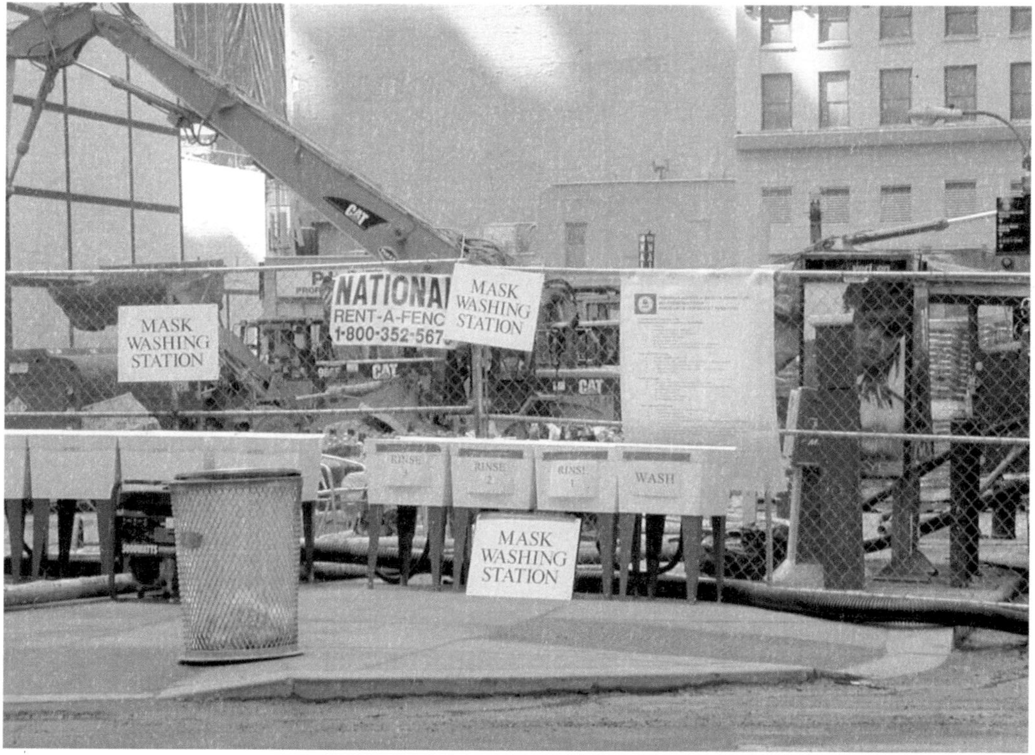

PHOTO 18. Abandoned Triage Station with Unused IV Bags Showing Un-abandoned Hope.

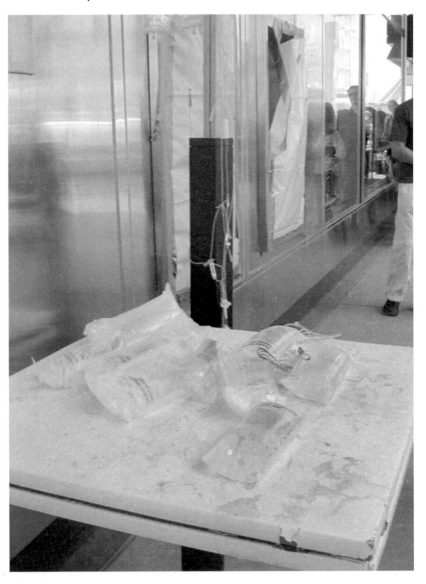

Photo by Donna Brennan. Used by permission.

PHOTO 19. Unused Medical Supplies Remain Taped to a Pole at Ground Zero Months After September 11th, 2001.

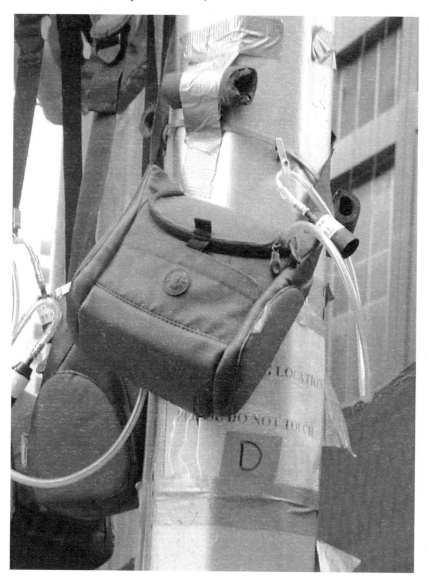

Photo by Donna Brennan. Used by permission.

Jane Prawda, an Occupational Therapist, further describes the Ground Zero milieu through her interview with the Chief of Battalion 50 of Queens, New York, and firefighter, Paul Tauber.

* * *

At the time of September 11th, 2001, Paul Tauber had been on the fire-fighting force for 23 years and was in charge of ten companies. He first learned of the plane crash while watching television. After viewing the news, he stated that he "already knew one hundred firefighters would be dead." He immediately called his battalion and rushed to Ground Zero, arriving shortly after the second tower fell. Tauber reported that other firefighters rushed to the site, taking passengers off public buses and commandeering the buses in order to make their way through the chaos.

Tauber's first reaction upon viewing the site of disaster was, *This is unbelievable.* He stated that he "must have repeated, *I cannot believe it* at least one hundred times" during his recovery work at Ground Zero that day and into the next morning. His co-worker, Battalion Chief Orio Palmer, was missing. Tauber knew he was dead.

In the aftermath of 9/11, Tauber described the Ground Zero milieu. He stated, "There was no time to process what was taking place. We would pick up things that did not look human. *Do your job* was always on my mind." He kept telling himself, *Do not give up, ever.* Although the firefighters were always under control, Tauber sensed feelings of hopelessness in his crew. He also noticed depression, numbing, increased arousal, avoidance, a state of shock and horror, and a significant amount of stress among his workers while on the job.

While off the job, Tauber commented that the firefighters were attending funerals. They worked on "autopilot" going from funeral to Ground Zero to funeral. Alcohol was prevalent at these funerals and was consumed as part of custom and also to relieve stress. As a result, many of the firefighters developed a drinking problem. Many had problems controlling their anger. Tauber commented that "the aftermath of [working at] Ground Zero is that nobody is the same." Professional counseling continues to be offered to date, free of charge, but most firefighters refuse it. Tauber asserts that this is "the John Wayne Syndrome"; indicating that the firefighters would prefer to be stoic, tough and continue to work rather than to seek help.

On September 11, 2001, 343 firefighters died. Tauber knew 280 of them. Eleven months later he admits that he is moved to tears whenever he encounters a symbol of American patriotism and cries when he experiences a trigger that reminds him of the event. Given all of the above, Paul Tauber expressed the sentiment that he and the rest of the firefighters "would rather die in the process of saving somebody" [than die in any other way].

* * *

These two narratives describing the Ground Zero milieu highlight the selfless acts of the firefighters who put the needs of others before their own. One can only imagine the enormous impact that this disaster had on firefighters who were reluctant to seek help for themselves. In the next chapter, a firefighter, in an attempt to relieve his emotional pain, begins to confide to his friend, an occupational therapist, about his experiences working at Ground Zero. Search and Rescue dogs, Veterinarians and Junior Firefighters were also part of the Ground Zero milieu as described in "The K-9 Unit" chapter. Due to the severe devastation, many occupational and physical therapists' businesses in lower Manhattan became inoperable. The Downtown Therapists Assistance Project as described in Iris Kimberg's chapter was started to help these NYC therapists become reestablished in the community. A section on the Ground Zero Milieu would not be complete without the inclusion of the Federal Emergency Management Agency and the role that an occupational therapy intern had in working within their Project Liberty. The final chapter of Section II analyzes the symptoms, responses, coping mechanisms and various interventions of/with two people who were present at Ground Zero on 9/11/2001.

Biography of a Ground Zero Firefighter

Mary Squillace, BA, BS/MS, OTR/L

In the wake of their immediate grief, survivors and others affected by this disaster are likely to be preoccupied with bringing the perpetrators to justice. They may find it hard to let go and rebuild their own lives. Rescue workers may face special emotional challenges. Usually they spend most of their time rescuing people who are alive; much of their professional identity is based on this fact. For them, this experience in which they have had to recover many dead victims may seem to be a personal failure. (Advance Online, 2002)

Billy is a New York City firefighter from Firehouse Engine 292 and Rescue 4. Rescue 4 was one of the first companies to respond to the World Trade Center site. Billy has been a personal friend of mine for many years. Because of our busy schedules, we had not spoken for some time. When this disaster occurred, I knew that there was a good chance that Billy would be at the site. I also knew that it would be difficult to contact him if he were alive. I waited until the next day and then went online to find a missing persons' list. Thankfully, Billy was not on that list. As time passed, I received a call from Billy. I had left several messages at the firehouse and he was returning my call. Hearing his familiar voice overwhelmed me with happiness. He said he called me because he needed to talk to someone. He said that although a therapist comes to the firehouse to speak with the men on an individual basis, he

---

[Haworth co-indexing entry note]: "Biography of a Ground Zero Firefighter." Squillace, Mary. Co-published simultaneously in *Occupational Therapy in Mental Health* (The Haworth Press, Inc.) Vol. 19, No. 3/4, 2003, pp. 103-114; and: *Surviving 9/11: Impact and Experiences of Occupational Therapy Practitioners* (ed: Pat Precin) The Haworth Press, Inc., 2003, pp. 103-114. Single or multiple copies of this article are available for a fee from The Haworth Document Delivery Service [1-800-HAWORTH, 9:00 a.m. - 5:00 p.m. (EST). E-mail address: docdelivery@haworthpress.com].

http://www.haworthpress.com/web/OTMH
Digital Object Identifier: 10.1300/J004v19n03_09

felt more comfortable speaking with a friend about his ordeal. I told him that I was available to listen to him and then advised him that, in the meanwhile, it would be a good idea for him to make an appointment with the current therapist that was at the firehouse.

I went to the firehouse and met with Billy. Several of the firefighters were present and very welcoming. I sat with Billy and listened to his stories. They were compelling and distressing and he appeared fatigued. I could see his sorrow, and, at the same time, I witnessed his ability to maintain control of his disposition. This is something that is assumed to be of second nature to someone who is faced with tragedy on a regular basis.

Billy's firehouse has suffered devastating losses. Just a few months before September 11th, Billy's firehouse lost two of their brothers in a fatal fire on Father's Day. Then on the infamous day of tragedy, firehouse engine 292 lost nine more brothers. Fortunately, Billy was off that day and was called by one of the firefighters about what had happened. Instinctually, Billy drove to the site to help his brothers. Upon his arrival, both towers had already collapsed and debris was widespread (Photos 1-7). He remembers standing in awe for some time before he could begin working. Billy recalls, "I felt helpless. There were so many beams, and they were approximately 18 tons each. I thought at first that we could save a lot of lives, but when I saw how bad this was, I knew we had suffered a great loss." Once he was given a briefing at Ground Zero, he began working. He admits that from the start of his work he became so obsessed with rescuing possible survivors that he could not stop working. He worked almost 24 hours a day for two months straight. There was little time for breaks because, according to Billy, there was always a sense that someone was alive in the debris.

As time passed, the hope began to diminish. Billy accepted the fact that those who survived this tragedy were already saved and there was no hope for more survivors. He states, "We were picking up body parts everyday. Heads, legs, fingers, and torsos, but rarely did we find intact bodies." He continues, "At first, it was discouraging to constantly pick up only parts, and after a while it stopped upsetting me. I realized that I was becoming numb to what would have been horrible to others. That is when I knew that I had to stop working and it was time to go home."

Billy admits to neglecting his own family and responsibilities during this time. He became so focused on saving lives that his own life was suffering. So he stopped. He states that he has developed a greater appreciation for his family and his own life.

PHOTO 1. Ground Zero.

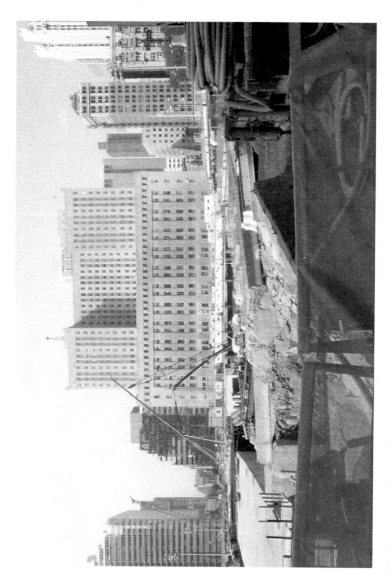

Photo by Pat Precin. Used by permission.

PHOTO 2. Ground Zero Below Street Level.

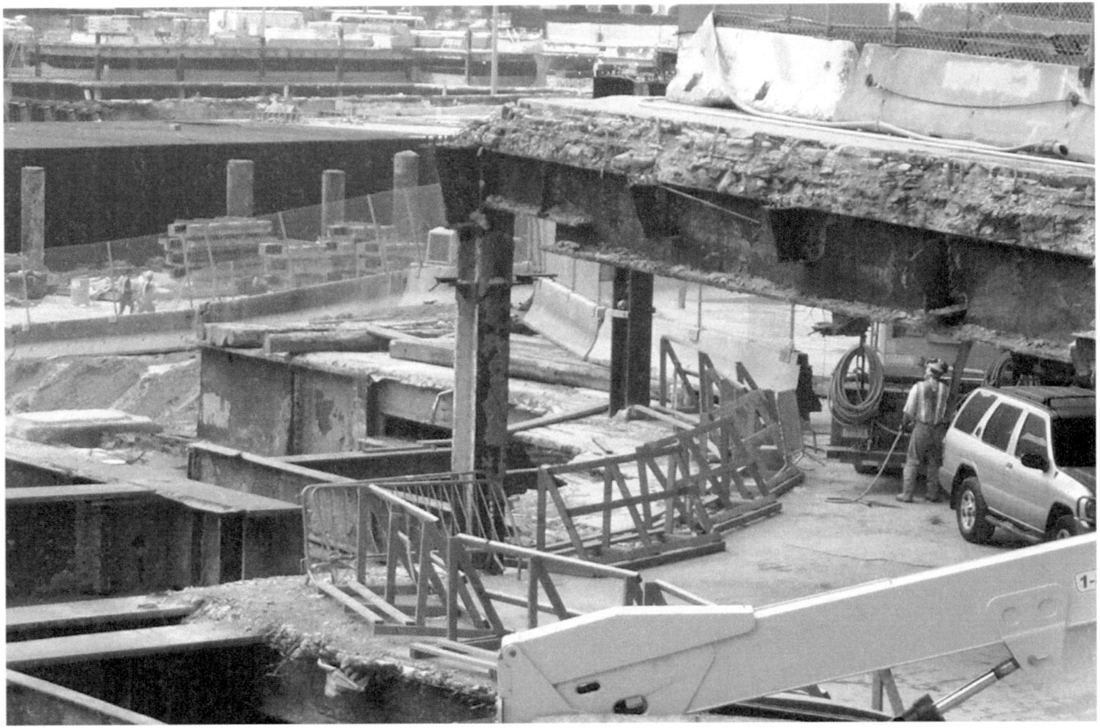

Photo by Pat Precin. Used by permission.

PHOTO 3. Ground Zero–Chunks of Exposed Concrete and Steel Reinforcers.

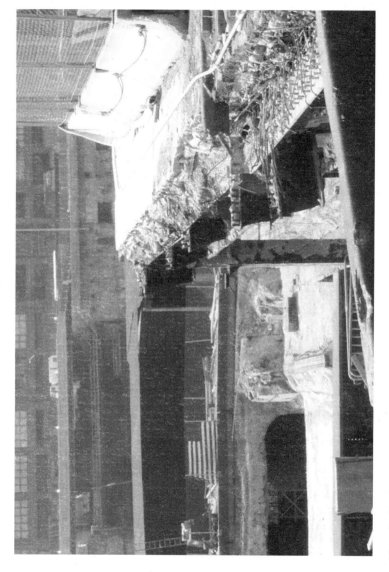

Photo by Pat Precin. Used by permission.

PHOTO 4. The Side of the Once World Trade Tower.

Photo by Pat Precin. Used by permission.

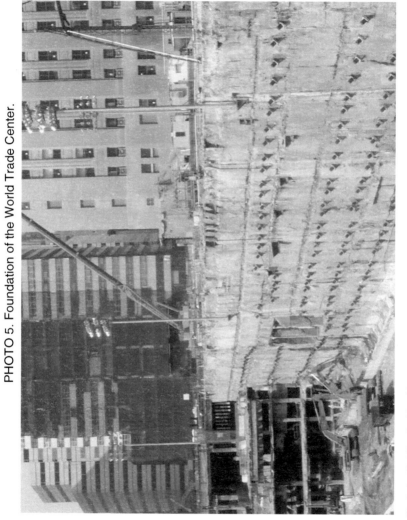

PHOTO 5. Foundation of the World Trade Center.

Photo by Pat Precin. Used by permission.

PHOTO 6. Holes or Wholes? It Is Up to Each of Us.

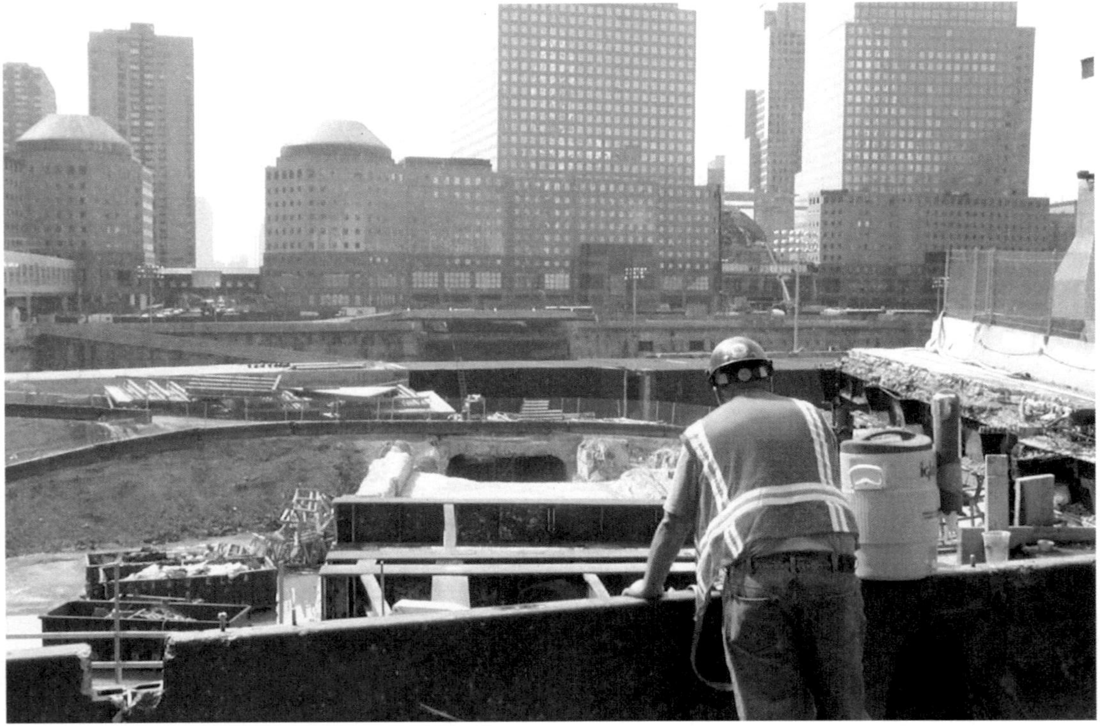

Photo by Pat Precin. Used by permission.

PHOTO 7. Collateral Damage. Nearby Buildings That Survived the Impact Are Draped in Construction Cloth Awaiting Treatments.

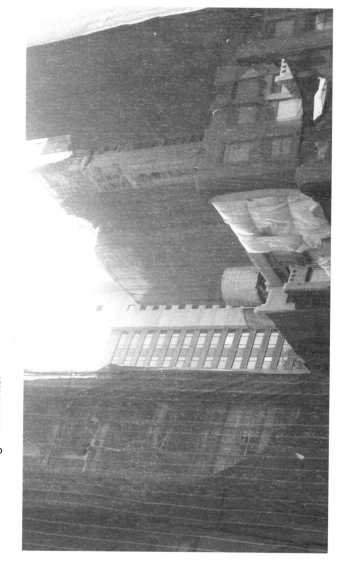

Photo by Pat Precin. Used by permission.

I asked if he becomes nervous upon every call for an emergency. He states, "You cannot think that every time you go out there that you are going to lose someone or possibly die. Yes, we keep in our heads that there is a possibility, and we are concerned about what we are about to be faced with, but our job is what it is, and we have to face the fire, so to speak, and worry later. We are used to feeling a little fearful with every run."

Billy told me that the men in the firehouse continue to maintain close relationships with the wives of the lost brothers. He states that many of the men are in a terrible state of mind and because of this, their lives have been affected as a whole. Some are experiencing marital difficulties and some are battling depression. Billy had been to the funerals and memorial services of many firefighters that were lost on that day and feels he has become hardened with emotion. He states that he breaks down at these services, especially when he sees the children of these men. He reflects on his own children and how he was lucky to have been off that day.

Regarding what could be done to help these men overcome the horrendous pain and anguish that they experienced, I first considered only positive ideas. I thought of what would create contentment for these men. The three ideas that surpassed all others were (1) develop a food group within the firehouse with just the firefighters, since these men love to cook; (2) organize a feast or picnic for the firefighters and their families at the firehouse or in a local park and; (3) offer hand massages for those who had worked hard that day. When I presented these ideas to Billy, he laughed. He stated that they already have many cooks in the house, including himself, and that these men can cook better than some of the best chefs in New York City. He continued to say that there is a picnic planned for the firefighters and their families annually. He then agreed that the hand massages was a good idea and that I could start with his hands.

The men at the firehouse have had much support from the New York City communities. Many people have offered their condolences by bringing food for the men and volunteering their time to run errands (Photo 8). They greatly appreciate the outpouring of love and concern. Billy states, "The community gave us the best therapy we could ever have. The love and support we received was tremendous and helped us through many hard times."

To some, returning to the workforce was a break from the reality of the events of 9/11. For Billy, facing this tragedy on a daily basis was his work. He was able to focus on the rescue efforts and not dwell on the travesty. It was when he realized that he was without emotional re-

PHOTO 8. Volunteers at the Salvation Army at 14th Street in Manhattan.

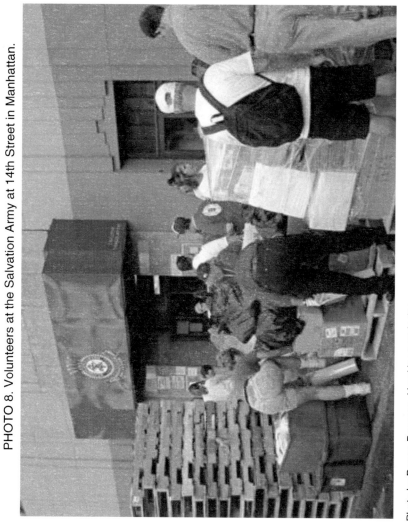

Photo by Donna Brennan. Used by permission.

sources during these efforts and he began feeling stoic that he relinquished his duties at the World Trade Center site. His grieving became apparent once he returned to his family and then to the firehouse where he realized his friends were no longer returning to work. "I cannot say that I am a stronger person from what I experienced, but I do know that anything is possible at this time and I am ready to face whatever is brought my way."

REFERENCE

Advance Online: National News. (2002). National News. *HHS addresses emotional and mental health consequences of attacks*. Retrieved June 14, 2002 from http://www.newsadvance.com

The K-9 Unit

Pat Precin, MS, OTR/L
Brad Gottlieb

After the September 11th disaster, people of all ages, cultures, professions, economic statuses, and religions mobilized to help people who were affected; in some way everyone was affected. Volunteering, working, or lending a hand not only helped victims but was also therapeutic for those providing services. This type of work provided some with a sense of purpose and structure in an otherwise unknown, out-of-control situation. Anger, rage, sorrow, anxiety, and other feelings otherwise overwhelming could be channeled in a dignified, positive way. Seeing others helping raised a sense of collective consciousness of hope, courage, and bravery necessary to carry people through.

But people were not the only ones helping. Dogs were helping, too. At times, they exhibited just as much courage, bravery, resilience, hard work and tenacity as humans. They, too, seem to benefit from a job well done. Any dog lover will agree that these animals need to feel useful on a regular basis, whether it is protecting the family, providing love, herding sheep, assisting people with disabilities, retrieving birds, or engaging in search and rescue at Ground Zero.

The following is a true story of dogs and people working together at Ground Zero relayed by the second author as he describes his work with the 9/11 K-9 Unit (canine unit) immediately following September 11th.

* * *

[Haworth co-indexing entry note]: "The K-9 Unit." Precin, Pat, and Brad Gottlieb. Co-published simultaneously in *Occupational Therapy in Mental Health* (The Haworth Press, Inc.) Vol. 19, No. 3/4, 2003, pp. 115-123; and: *Surviving 9/11: Impact and Experiences of Occupational Therapy Practitioners* (ed: Pat Precin) The Haworth Press, Inc., 2003, pp. 115-123. Single or multiple copies of this article are available for a fee from The Haworth Document Delivery Service [1-800-HAWORTH, 9:00 a.m. - 5:00 p.m. (EST). E-mail address: docdelivery@haworthpress.com].

Digital Object Identifier: 10.1300/J004v19n03_10

115

It started out as a normal day typical for September, breezy and pleasant. My friend, Justin, and I had just finished our second period class and decided to run across the street from the High School to grab a bagel and orange juice at the local deli. When we entered, we happened to glance at the television and saw what we thought was a disaster movie. On the screen was an image of one of the Twin Towers on fire. We stood on line for our breakfast, sat down, and continued to watch the "movie." Suddenly, when a plane struck the second tower, fiction became fact and we realized that the images on the screen were those of America under attack. At that moment, our emergency pagers sounded, and the dispatcher came on and said, "All available manpower report to the Firehouse." As a volunteer Junior Firefighter since 1997, I knew that I needed to respond and go to the firehouse. What I did not know at that moment was how profoundly my life would change as a result of September 11th.

Around the clock for the next forty-eight hours, all of the junior firefighters at the Hewlett Fire House served as errand runners, messengers, standby crew, as "extra muscle." All the senior firefighters from the local towns were pulled into Manhattan, leaving the junior firefighters as the skeletal/standby crew, who faced the possibility of having to answer local fire calls. Later that evening, our chief held a meeting to discuss our responsibilities if and when there was an additional threat or attack. Although the five of us who remained were frightened, each of us wanted to be able to go to Ground Zero to give more than we were giving now. It was the moment I returned home exhausted on September 12th at midnight that I realized my desire to help more might be realized.

When I arrived home that night, I found out that my father, who is a veterinarian, had been called by the Suffolk County American Society for the Prevention of Cruelty to Animals (ASPCA) to go to Ground Zero and volunteer his services for the K-9 Search and Rescue dogs. When I asked my father if I could accompany him, my mother was reluctant to let both of us go. My father and I have always been a team, and ever since I can remember, I have always loved animals and wanted to be a veterinarian. I explained to my mother that since so many people were in pain, if we could help in any way, this would be our chance to comfort those feeling the effects of the attack. My mother understood and unenthusiastically agreed to let us go.

I woke up the next morning at 5:00 a.m. to find my father packing a full carload of veterinary supplies. We left for Ground Zero at about 5:30 a.m. and arrived at 6:45 a.m., after going through extensive police blockades and checkpoints. We unloaded the car, and walked six blocks to the horrendous site of the collapsed Twin Towers, only to arrive at one of the most difficult and unforgettable events of my life. Before I put on the surgical mask, I smelled death in the dust-filled air. As I got closer to Ground Zero I noticed that normal city buildings had become heaps of twisted metal covered with a shroud of fiberglass/plaster "snow." We made our way to a tent labeled, "Suffolk County ASPCA/VMAT." We were working with the ASPCA and Veterinary Medical Assistance Teams.

When we got settled, five veterinarians started to explain to us what they needed and how we were to go about taking care of the cadaver dogs (Photo 1). These are dogs that specialize in sniffing for bodies and body parts. They were mostly Labrador retrievers, which are known for their excellent temperaments. Most of them had previously worked for the Police K-9 unit. Both dogs and people came from all over the United States and Canada and Europe. When the dogs came from the fifteen-story pile of debris, we first had to wash all their fur. Dogs find parts of bodies by scent; after working in the "pile" for some time they must be cleansed of the smoke and other odors from the fire so they can return to their job at the pile. Our second duty was to make sure that they had not hurt their paws (Photo 2). This was important because the dogs were walking across the pieces of steel and metal that were extremely hot. The dogs were equipped with little booties to keep their paws from burning. Most of the search and rescue dogs did not like them and we were forced to take them off. In addition to paw maintenance, attention to skin and fur hygiene was critical in maintaining a healthy animal as pieces of debris can cause skin irritations and singed fur. Our third responsibility was to re-hydrate the dogs. Most of the dogs were lethargic and did not want any water so we had to give them intravenous fluids. The dogs would work on twelve-hour shifts, about five dogs and trainers would be on the "pile" at a time. Their trainer would follow directly behind them and when a dog would locate a body part they would sit down or start to bark. It was very upsetting because when the dogs came off of the "pile" they were extremely tired and would collapse when we started to take care of them. The veterinarian (my father) would make sure their vital signs were normal.

When I was working on the dogs, I noticed that their demeanor, like mine, was one of grief but determination. Like the dogs, I was standing in the midst of a devastation so enormous that I could not take it all in at once. In some ways, dogs are like humans; they get very frustrated when they do not make a find (find a human body or part). The dogs work on a reward system: when they find something, they receive praise and a biscuit. The veterinarians had decided to set up a mock situation in which the dogs would go into a building down the street and find a fake

PHOTO 1. A German Shepherd Cadaver Dog.

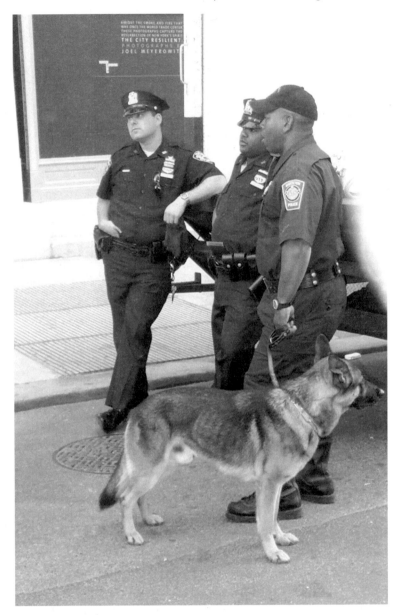

Photo by Pat Precin. Used by permission.

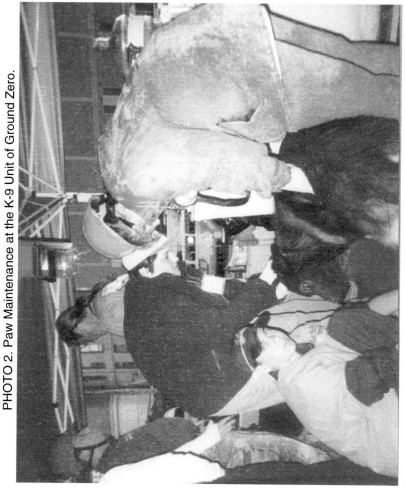

PHOTO 2. Paw Maintenance at the K-9 Unit of Ground Zero.

Photo by Dr. Jay Gottlieb. Used by permission.

victim. This "find" would boost the animal's confidence and also let the animal know that it was doing the right thing. I had worked at Ground Zero for two days straight with no sleep. The dogs, however, worked incessantly for weeks and when these canine heroes were pulled away from the pile of debris, I knew I wanted to devote my life to working with animals!

It is almost a cliché to talk about the impact that September 11th has had on people. My story is just one of many stories; I did not lose anyone in the attack, so I cannot speak about that kind of grief. The attacks left me full of anger, helplessness, and frustration, but at the same time I felt pride in the efforts of all the good people and K-9 Unit around me. September 11 put things in perspective for me. I learned that dogs are like humans and that we must treat them in a humane way. It reaffirmed my love for animals (dogs are indeed our best friend) and my commitment to helping others by serving my community. Unfortunately, it took a disaster to bring the nation closer together and make me realize how precious and fragile life can be at times. It also made me more determined to not let my learning disabilities get in the way of reaching my dreams. Many people who perished in the attacks probably did not live long enough to reach all of their goals in life. So now I cherish my goal of becoming a veterinarian even more.

* * *

In the narrative above, Brad shares his aspiration to become a veterinarian, but he already possesses many characteristics of a good occupational therapist as demonstrated by his work with the canines. He performed activities of daily living (ADLs) for them: washing their fur, mending their paws, checking their skin, and providing intravenous fluid replacement. Through acute observation skills and sensitivity, he assessed the canines' overall mental status to be one of grief, determination, and by the end of the day, lethargy. He encouraged their work by using biscuits as a positive reward. He even graded the activity of search and rescue by creating a "mock find" in another nearby building because the lack of "finds" at Ground Zero was causing the canines to become discouraged. He demonstrated empathy with this discouragement by relating it to human discouragement experienced under the same circumstances. These "mock finds" increased the canines' confidence levels and reinforced positive behaviors. His work was emotionally and physically demanding (as is much of our work as occupational therapists), yet he was able to continue in an effective way for forty-eight hours straight. Brad was able to focus his feelings of anger, helplessness and frustration into meaningful activity and felt pride in doing so, a pride that allowed him to learn from this devastating experience. He re-affirmed his love for animals, community work, and the preciousness of life. He took these affirmations and set a goal to never let his learning disabilities get in the way of achieving his personal goal of becoming a veterinarian.

In honor of the K-9 Unit, sculptures of search and rescue dogs were created and displayed in various parts of New York City under the title of "DOGNY–America's Tribute to Search and Rescue Dogs" (Photos 3-5).

PHOTO 3. Sculpture of Search and Rescue Dog "Rushing to the Rescue" by Artist Claudia Nagy.

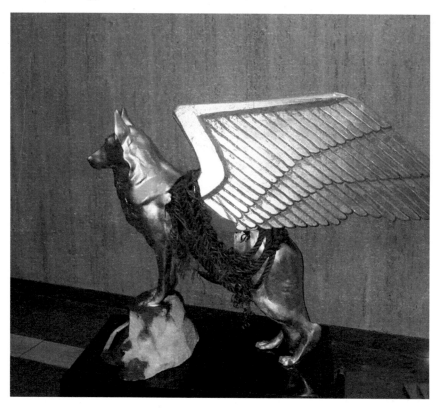

Photo by Pat Precin. Used by permission.

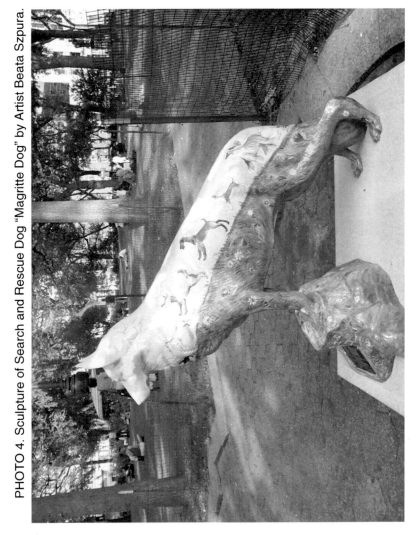

PHOTO 4. Sculpture of Search and Rescue Dog "Magritte Dog" by Artist Beata Szpura.

Photo by Pat Precin. Used by permission.

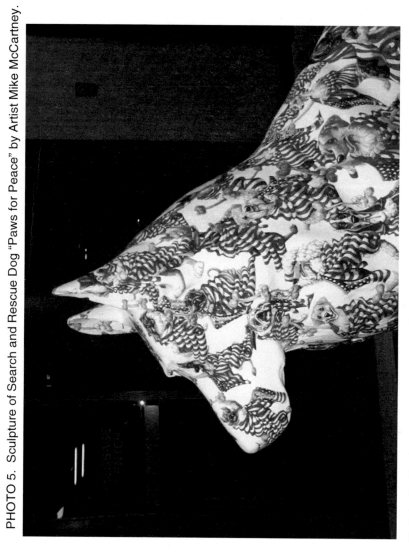

PHOTO 5. Sculpture of Search and Rescue Dog "Paws for Peace" by Artist Mike McCartney.

Photo by Pat Precin. Used by permission.

The Downtown
Therapists' Assistance Project

Iris Kimberg, MS, PT, OTR

Tribeca, located in downtown New York, has been my home for the last twenty-five years. It is where I raised my daughter Jenna, now thirteen, and where I have practiced both as an occupational and a physical therapist in many business ventures since 1979. The events of September 11th impacted me as they did everyone else; on many different levels, and in many ways. Having this happen in my own neighborhood was especially challenging: I saw the disaster, I smelled the disaster, and I lived in it day after day. At first my world was consumed by day-to-day survival: identification cards were needed to gain access below Canal Street, no personal vehicles were allowed in, and there were no means of reliable public transportation or open stores for daily food. Day by day, I would wait to hear from neighbors and friends to see who needed what, be it a place to stay, a meal, or just a familiar shoulder to cry on. I did what I could to help my neighbors and my neighborhood survive: going to the make-shift food kitchens, handing out face masks, giving water to the rescue dogs as they marched along Hudson Street.

I began to wonder how all the therapy practices in the downtown vicinity were surviving. Being both an occupational therapist and a physical therapist and having been downtown for so long, I knew almost all of the practices, some superficially and some intimately. Most were well-known, long-established practices, owned by solo practitioners.

[Haworth co-indexing entry note]: "The Downtown Therapists' Assistance Project." Kimberg, Iris. Co-published simultaneously in *Occupational Therapy in Mental Health* (The Haworth Press, Inc.) Vol. 19, No. 3/4, 2003, pp. 125-127; and: *Surviving 9/11: Impact and Experiences of Occupational Therapy Practitioners* (ed: Pat Precin) The Haworth Press, Inc., 2003, pp. 125-127. Single or multiple copies of this article are available for a fee from The Haworth Document Delivery Service [1-800-HAWORTH, 9:00 a.m. - 5:00 p.m. (EST). E-mail address: docdelivery@haworthpress.com].

http://www.haworthpress.com/web/OTMH
Digital Object Identifier: 10.1300/J004v19n03_11

As phone service began to be restored in the area, I started an informal fact-finding mission, contacting the fourteen practices I was aware of, either by phone if possible, or mail if not. Needless to say, all were impacted by the disastrous events of 9/11. Thankfully, all the therapists were able to evacuate their offices along with their early morning patients, including a therapist who had a corporate branch of her practice in the World Trade Center Hotel.

One occupational therapy practice, located within a half of a block of the World Trade Center, was owned by a close personal friend, Susan Scanga, MA, OTR, CHT. Her office, part of a loft where she also lived for over twenty years, sustained extensive internal damage from fallen debris/ash and as of August 2002, remains completely shut down. In January of 2002, Susan relocated to a new temporary home where she has again begun treating patients on a part-time basis, while still awaiting word on whether she will ever be able to return to her original home and office.

A physical therapy practice owned by a former classmate of mine was located one block from the World Trade Center. His practice remained closed until mid-November, when the police re-opened his block to the general public. Travel to the area of his practice remained severely restricted until the clean-up of the World Trade Center was complete. It also became apparent that much of his client base was businesses that had been forced to relocate, most of them uptown.

Another practice hard hit was a pediatric practice owned by Linda Rowe, registered occupational therapist. Located four blocks north of the World Trade Center, her office remained closed for weeks while she awaited the specialized environmental cleaning and attempted to replace the equipment that she needed. When she did re-open, it was with a reduced staff and a much smaller caseload; many of her clients' families lived locally and were displaced to other areas of Manhattan. Other clients were reluctant to come back to the area, especially those with high-risk babies, because of lingering air quality concerns. In addition, many of her pre-school and school-aged clients had to make arrangements with other practices uptown since she was closed for so many weeks.

It did not take long for me to realize that these practices were hard hit by the events of 9/11–psychologically, physically and economically. After talking to these business owners/therapists, I realized that they, like most therapists, did not like to ask for help even though they needed it. That, combined with my own desire as a therapist to help, led me to organize the Downtown Therapists' Assistance Project (DNAP). I knew that there were other therapists like myself out there who wanted to help. Within a week, the fund was up and running, and as word of it spread, so did the financial and emotional support from therapists and vendors across the country.

Jenna was in charge of opening the mail that started to come in. How exciting it was for her to see mail from as close as Brooklyn, New York, to as far away as Soquel, California. Donations of $14.00 from a certified occupational therapy assistant program in Mississippi were as important to us as the $10,000 in equipment from Smith and Nephew, Inc. An occupational therapy department in New Jersey contributed money normally used for a Christmas buffet. A hand therapy practice in Vermont sent a contribution instead of gifts normally given to referring physicians. The Massachusetts Association for Occupational Therapy, and the American Society of Hand Therapists both raised funds for DTAP during their annual meetings. One therapist from Ohio flew to New York to personally bring a donation and come see the destruction for herself. Both the local and national occupational therapy and physical therapy Associations helped to publicize the fund on their Web sites.

All in all, therapists, hospitals, private practices and equipment vendors from twenty-eight states contributed in excess of $25,000 in money and equipment, with 100% of the proceeds going directly to the therapists in need. Almost all of the donations were accompanied by personal handwritten notes of love, support and encouragement. Jenna asked how long we should keep the fund going. The answer is easy: until the last therapist is back in her office. Donations can still be made to:

Downtown Therapists' Assistance Project (DNAP)
c/o Iris Kimberg, MS, PT, OTR
105 Hudson Street 11N
NY, NY 10013

(Updates on the fund and therapists are posted at *www. nytherapyguide.com*)

Coping with Tragedy:
A Fieldwork Student's Experience
with FEMA Crisis Counseling

Jennifer Persh, MA, OTR

I had just started my second Level II Fieldwork placement at a homeless shelter and mental health clinic at the beginning of September 2001. During this mental health affiliation, I worked with another student to provide occupational therapy services to residents of the shelter and clients of the clinic. Our main goal at this fieldwork was to develop a new life skills program for the clients, which was to consist of daily groups tailored around their needs. As we were just starting to get to know the clients and to understand the workings of this complex downtown shelter and clinic, the September eleventh attacks occurred. That day, I was supposed to arrive and stay late in order to lead nightly activities. I never made it in that day, or for the rest of the week.

On that fateful Tuesday morning, I was awakened by a call from my aunt in California who wanted to make sure I was not affected by the attacks. Like everyone else in the world, I was stunned. When I got over the initial shock of what had happened, I wondered what was happening at the shelter. Most of the residents were without social supports. Who would they talk to? I was worried about my friends and family, and I was hoping that they had someone to help them as well. Many of the clients of the clinic live in downtown Manhattan. Would they still be able to travel to get to their doctor's appointments, buy food, or fill prescrip-

[Haworth co-indexing entry note]: "Coping with Tragedy: A Fieldwork Student's Experience with FEMA Crisis Counseling." Persh, Jennifer. Co-published simultaneously in *Occupational Therapy in Mental Health* (The Haworth Press, Inc.) Vol. 19, No. 3/4, 2003, pp. 129-143; and: *Surviving 9/11: Impact and Experiences of Occupational Therapy Practitioners* (ed: Pat Precin) The Haworth Press, Inc., 2003, pp. 129-143. Single or multiple copies of this article are available for a fee from The Haworth Document Delivery Service [1-800-HAWORTH, 9:00 a.m. - 5:00 p.m. (EST). E-mail address: docdelivery@haworthpress.com].

http://www.haworthpress.com/web/OTMH
Digital Object Identifier: 10.1300/J004v19n03_12

tions? What makes this population unique is that in order to qualify to receive services, the clients must have a physical disability. Because of this, many of them have limitations in terms of their mobility and require daily medications in order to maintain their health. New York City had shut down. Were they still able to get what they needed to survive?

When I returned to the shelter on the following Monday, the atmosphere was quiet and tense. I still did not know the residents very well and I was nervous that I would never get to know them under these circumstances. The other student and I decided that we would try during an activity to get the residents to discuss what had happened. A previous student at the shelter had informed us that the residents loved to work on art and crafts projects, so we brought down some materials to create patriotic crafts. In school, I had just learned about the impact of activity on a person's ability to express his or her emotions. I was now able to see this firsthand.

We sat outside on the patio gluing and painting American flags made out of Popsicle sticks. As we did this, the clients, who never even knew us, started freely expressing their feelings. I distinctly remember one woman breaking down in tears. Emma was a clinically depressed woman who believed that these terrorist attacks marked the end of the world. At the time of the tragedy, she did not have contact with anyone in her family. Emma's one support, her grandmother, had just passed away. She was alone and now she was terrified that the world was going to end. She could barely bring herself to pick up any of the materials and spent the entire session crying. John was also seated at the table. An outspoken man, he began to yell at Emma, speaking about the politics of the tragedy and how the United States must take immediate action. It was not that they were on different sides; he was just angry and began to yell at the easiest target.[1]

Being a student, just starting a new fieldwork, I was confused about how to handle this situation. Emma would not defend herself. She remained quiet and seated while John yelled at her. John would not give up, despite being told by the other student, the residents, and I to stop. After a few minutes the argument ended. Later, we addressed this in our small informal groups. We discussed that tragedies often bring out the best and the worst in people. On one hand, we must remember that tragedies such as this create tremendous amounts of stress, even for people who were not directly involved. Some people handle stress by taking it out on others. However, the group agreed that this was not an effective means of coping. On the other hand, one resident believed that people need to defend themselves. It is acceptable to get up and leave or to speak back in a polite, yet firm manner. This then led to numerous groups on the topic of communication skills, and how to use verbal and non-verbal ways to communicate points of view in an acceptable manner.

After the first few days, it was evident that everyone at the shelter was affected by the attacks. It soon became clear that many of the missing family and friends of employees and clients were not going to be found. During the groups, many concerns were expressed. The first one was the desire to help. What I found so amazing was that I was working with people who were facing tremendous difficulties. The students of the shelter were disabled and had little money. Most had no social supports. However, as soon as the tradgedy happened, they immediately went to the nearby fire station that had lost many members to bring some food. They wanted to help others who were in need.

Every week, the occupational therapy students facilitated a community group that the clinic clients attended. It centered on advocacy and planning activities for the disabled community. During the weeks following the attacks, we discussed different ways that the group could contribute by helping victims of the attacks and their families. First, we discussed how people were affected. This allowed the members to express their feelings about the severity of the tragedy and to try to comprehend what happened. Then the members thought about people's needs and what could be done to meet these needs. The group members indicated that this activity let them feel a sense of control in that it gave them a goal to work towards in order to give something back to the community.

One concern was evident in all the groups. Coping with the unknown of what exactly happened to those who were missing and accepting their death, even for people who had not lost anyone, was difficult to work through. The hardest part was that most of the residents were not able to easily communicate with their friends and families. Many of them had not spoken to their families in years and they had no idea where their loved ones were living. One woman, Sarah, swore her dad was killed. It was extremely hard for her. Due to the fact that she had a psychiatric illness, she frequently provided false information concerning details of her life. We did not know if she was being accurate with her facts. If she was, how could she find out if he was alive, and how were we to help her get through this? If this did not turn out to be the truth, we wanted to help her work through the thought that led her to this belief.

New York was also dealing with the threat of additional terrorist attacks. This topic fit right into our life skills group series. Although the topics were not focused around the September eleventh attacks, the groups helped people to cope with the tragedy. The consumers receiving services at the clinic and shelter had special needs beyond the average person. Many of the consumers were visually impaired, deaf, and used crutches, walkers, or wheelchairs. Additionally, almost everyone depended on taking daily medications. This means they needed to get to the nearby pharmacy every month. During these attacks, most businesses closed for several days. Everyone expressed anxiety that if this happened again for longer periods, their physical and mental health would suffer from not having access to their medications. Additionally, the World Trade Center once stood only blocks away from the shelter and they were scared that they could be the victims of another direct attack. They worried about other things as well. With a sensory impairment, many people may not be aware of an emergency if they cannot hear or see alarms. Even if they were aware of an attack, how would they escape down the stairs in an emergency situation? As a group, we problem solved different methods to cope with these fears. The most effective strategy was to determine actual strategies to employ, such as packing away extra clothes, some money, and a week's worth of medications in a safe place. We discussed that it is important to update this emergency kit to ensure the medications do not expire. We also talked about establishing a meeting place, such as specific emergency shelters or a family or friend's home if possible.

Although the groups helped the consumers to cope in practical ways, the media constantly played images of the past events. The threat of future attacks was clear and anthrax was in the process of claiming several lives in New York City and the surrounding areas. Some consumers found themselves compulsively reading the newspapers and watching television in order to obtain more information. This prevented them from completing their daily tasks and from taking part in leisure activities being held in and around the shelter. Often, just as consumers were able to separate themselves from the media, the government would issue another terrorist warning and the cycle would start again. It was a challenge to motivate some of the clients to attend our groups when they had something else keeping their minds busy. During the groups, I found that everyone had their own views on the media. Some needed to watch television, listen to the radio, and read the newspaper to put their minds at ease. When they did not have access to information, they felt uneasy and worried. Others said that they could not hear or read anything more, as the information was too distressing. As an occupational therapy student, I had to respect that everyone has his or her own way of coping. I could only stress that whatever consumers did, they must ensure that they were taking care of their own health and finding time to enjoy themselves in addition to how they spend the rest of their time.

Groups and informal conversations assisted the residents and clients in moving on from this tragedy, however, one event held at the shelter allowed the clients to feel a sense of closure. The shelter held a day of remembrance. This consisted of an hour-long ceremony in which employees and consumers were given a chance to speak about the tragedy. This service had a significant impact on the consumers in that everyone needed this event to be acknowledged formally. As in any death, people needed closure and this event served as a form of a funeral. It provided everyone an opportunity to say prayers for those who had passed or were still missing, and to acknowledge as a group that a horrible tragedy had occurred.

The occupational therapy program had a significant role in this ceremony. In the weeks before the event, we arranged for the consumers to make a large American flag and to cut out small stars. At the service, each consumer and employee wrote his or her name on a star. The stars were then attached to the flag, which remained on the cafeteria wall. This activity helped the consumers to have something concrete to remember the tragedy by. It provided them with a reference to look at that signified the tragedy and those who were lost.

It soon became obvious that most New Yorkers, even those that were not directly affected by the tragedy, were suffering. They were facing both practical problems, such as losing their homes and jobs, and emotional difficulties in dealing with the attacks. Therefore, during my experience at the shelter, the Federal Emergency Management Agency (FEMA) created a program called Project Liberty to assist New Yorkers in coping with the disaster. It was expected that over a million people were in need of mental health services in the New York City area and mental health agencies around New York were going to provide community outreach services to help anyone who required crisis counseling (Federal Emergency Management Agency, personal communication, October 11, 2001). In preparation for this event, I attended several disaster relief conferences and workshops that provided information and a chance to practice crisis-counseling techniques.

The Federal Emergency Management Agency presented one of these conferences and professionals from all disciplines attended the training. Other occupational therapists, social workers, nurses, and psychologists all came together to see how they could help. We received information regarding the structure of Project Liberty and specific counseling techniques.

The bombing in Oklahoma City was used as a model for the New York City attacks, as a similar program had been proven to be effective following their 1995 disaster. The Federal Emergency Management Agency structured Project Liberty in a way that they would teach New Yorkers how to help themselves. In order to do this, those in New York with a background in crisis counseling would train others. We were to work on teams consisting of at least one mental health professional, such as an individual with a master's degree in psychology, social work, counseling, or psychiatric nursing. Paraprofessionals and people indigenous to the community would also make up an essential part of the team (Center for Mental Health Services, 2000).

The program works in three stages. The first stage, that I took part in, was meant to offer short-term, practical, problem-solving techniques rather than intense psychological therapy. The counseling was to take place in common meeting centers, such as shelters or community centers, in order to find survivors and assess their needs in their own environment. The team of counselors was to first present a short information session regarding Project Liberty services in common meeting places such as places of worship or community centers. At this time, they could also train others, such as day care workers or guidance counselors on how to help people in need. Workers were to allow survivors to tell their stories and determine if they were in need of additional counseling. If called for, the individuals could then receive short-term crisis counseling in their home or in the community. The main goal of the counseling sessions would be to provide education about normal reactions and make referrals for long-term counseling if needed. Finally, the Project Liberty workers could also help with planning and implementing memorial events in the community (Center for Mental Health Services, 2000).

The Federal Emergency Management Agency designed this program based on several principles. The first important issue that was stressed is that most people do not seek out help following a disaster. Rather, many believe that others may need it more. Therefore, the outreach model is essential in providing needed services. This means going to places that New Yorkers may typically gather, such as in disaster centers, in their homes, or places of worship, is imperative for the program to be effective (Center for Mental Health Services, 2000). Besides this, a counselor should refrain from pressuring someone into accepting something they are not ready to come to terms with yet (Center for Mental Health

Services, 2000). For example, at this point, it was known that most of the missing individuals had been killed. However, many of their friends and family members were not ready to hold a funeral or memorial service. It is not the counselor's position to press the individual into holding such a service. Instead, it is best to wait for the person to be ready to carry through with the event. In addition to this, the counselor should help individuals understand that their reactions are most likely normal and help to bring back a sense of normalcy in their everyday lives (Center for Mental Health Services, 2000).

Counseling should also be flexible in helping the client deal with different issues in the setting where they are to function to deal with practical problems in addition to emotional or psychological impacts. The counselor should take on a role as a facilitator in helping the client to determine the most important issue and then solve this problem. Finally, just as in dealing in any other interaction, the counselor must take the individual's culture and religion into consideration and respect the corresponding rituals and practices (DeWolfe, 2000). Overall, the worker can provide both informal and formal counseling. The worker can look at the survivor's strengths and weaknesses, coping skills, and ways that the survivor has compensated for deficits over the past months in the environment that the survivor is now functioning in, then assist the survivor in initiating the healing process (Center for Mental Health Services, 2000).

Many techniques were provided to assist the counselor in providing effective services (DeWolfe, 2000). In the beginning, it is important to establish a trusting relationship by letting the individual know that the worker is there to help. Supportive listening allows a person to express thoughts regarding the event and how they have functioned since then (Federal Emergency Management Agency, personal communication, October 11, 2001). Provide the opportunity for the individual to first quietly consider his or her problems and then allow communication of these thoughts and feelings. In this way, information regarding this person's problems can be obtained. Some areas to work on may include re-establishing routines, providing opportunities to talk, assisting the individual in making contact with loved ones, and giving information about typical reactions and coping skills (DeWolfe, 2000). In order to assist the individual to solve problems on his or her own, the worker can provide appropriate resources to help the client create and implement a plan of action. The worker takes the consumer through the various steps necessary to address each issue (DeWolfe, 2000). The worker can also provide assistance to help the individual communicate with family members (DeWolfe, 2000).

Providing the consumer with coping strategies in order to increase his or her ability to deal with the tragedy is important. Some of these include avoiding excessive exposure to the media in the form of television, newspapers, and the radio. Looking at the bright side of the situation, such as how everyone was able to come together following the tragedy to help each other, is an important aspect of the disaster to keep in mind. Exploring activities that the client enjoys, such as hobbies or volunteering, can give the client a sense of purpose and a chance to think about things other than the disaster. Helping others who have been through this disaster or listening to people who have experienced a similar loss can help clients deal with their own emotions. The Counselor can also provide activities that help clients release anger, such as yoga, meditation, and exercise. Finally, explaining to the survivor that it is all right to allow others to help and to realize that many people experience similar feelings following a disaster can increase the survivor's ability to cope (American Red Cross in Greater New York, 2001).

Overall, the courses emphasized several areas of disaster mental health counseling that I needed to keep in mind when counseling clients. One key fact that was taught was that everyone who sees the tragedy is affected by it, whether it is seen on television or in person (DeWolfe, 2000). This means that just about everyone I would be coming across should have at least one issue that could be addressed. Following this is the concept that stress is a normal reaction as part of the grieving process. These reactions are often brought on by the everyday problems following a tragedy, such as transportation, accessing money, buying food, and obtaining medications (DeWolfe, 2000). In addition, the fact that there was no advanced warning and therefore the community could not prepare for a disaster influences the population's ability to deal with a disaster (Federal Emergency Management Agency, personal communication, October 11, 2001). Each client seeking services has factors that may influence his or her ability to deal with stress. Therefore, when addressing problems, it is important to examine one's ability to function in their environment. This includes access to resources, economic status, social supports, one's cognitive ability to understand what has happened and realistic future expectations (Federal Emergency Management Agency, personal communication, October 11, 2001).

The nature of the September eleventh events as a violent crime has specific qualities that influence a victim's ability to cope. This tragedy killed civilians on a large scale, was unexpected, and left people with a sense that they had no control over their environment. It violated their homes, places of employment, and impacted on every area of daily life. These factors are directly associated with depression, anxiety, and post-traumatic stress disorder that may last for long periods of time (Center for Mental Health Services, 2001). Besides the actual tragedy, the media's intense interest in replaying the events may have caused individuals to experience the trauma again through repeated exposure. The belief that a similar event may occur in the future may add to the already existing anxiety (American Red Cross in Greater New York, 2001).

Typical reactions can be expected following this type of disaster. Sources of problems include employment loss, family conflicts or losses, dealing with bureaucracies in order to achieve access to resources, the disruption that the process of cleaning up and rebuilding brings about, loss of support systems, and school closings and changes (Federal Emergency Management Agency, personal communication, October 11, 2001). Many will experience anxiety over additional practical problems such as relocating homes and places of employment, transportation changes, filling prescriptions, getting finances in order, and existing in a city at risk of being attacked again in the near future (DeWolfe, 2000).

Expected behavioral reactions to these problems may include problems falling or staying asleep, nightmares, avoiding reminders, an increased activity level without accomplishing the same amount of tasks, crying, withdrawal, avoidance or nervousness when traveling to certain places, and increased fighting with friends and family (DeWolfe, 2000). There are numerous physical reactions that are normal to experience following a disaster. These include changes in eating habits and appetite, fatigue, gastrointestinal system problems, and an increase in any chronic conditions that one may already have (DeWolfe, 2000). Typical psychological reactions may include depression, irritability, anxiety, guilt over surviving, self-doubt, and mood swings (DeWolfe, 2000). Persistent negative thoughts about the disaster or future events, recurring images and nightmares about the event, memory and concentration difficulties, confusion, disorientation, difficulty making decisions, the desire to constantly protect loved ones, and questioning of one's own spiritual beliefs are typical cognitive reactions to the disaster (Federal Emergency Management Agency, personal communication, October 11, 2001). Over time, some reactions may remain. One may continue to experience anxiety, anger, resentment, a decreased ability to problem-solve in common situations, health problems, uncertainty about the future, increased mourning of losses, isolation, hopelessness, depression, suicide thoughts and attempts, and alcohol and drug use to cope with these feelings (Federal Emergency Management Agency, personal communication, October 11, 2001). It is important to keep these common reactions in mind. In this way, the counselor can educate the client on normal reactions and intervene or provide referrals for further care if a reaction becomes severe.

Because my fieldwork facility serviced people with a mental illness and a physical disability, one aspect of the conferences that assisted me in my ability to provide crisis-counseling services was receiving information regarding those with mental illnesses and physical disabilities. Those with physical disabilities may experience additional anxiety because they may depend on others for their care and mobility. Any changes in their routine can cause a significant amount of stress. This may include changes in their physical environment (DeWolfe, 2000). Those with prior mental health illness have the same needs as the general population; however, outreach services are provided to help deal with medication needs, anxiety, or other symptoms of their disease that may be triggered by an event such as this (DeWolfe, 2000).

I was finally ready to begin counseling. In late November, I attended a presentation given by two of my Project Liberty team members at an apartment complex that houses people who have physical disabilities. From the beginning, it was obvious how upset the audience members had been since the tragedy. What started out as being a factual information session on the type of services that were to be available soon became an emotional group in which the audience members shared their fears and experiences. Overall, it was clear that they were terrified. Most of them were not involved in the tragedy; however, many people shared similar experiences they had been through and had not yet come to terms with. Furthermore, their current fears of additional terrorist attacks had been a great source of pain and stress since September eleventh.

Most of these people had needed someone to talk to, but they did not know where to go. This was in November, and the audience members believed that most of the acute counseling opportunities had passed. Very few of them were directly affected, but they still suffered and were not actively seeking help. Something so horrible had happened so close to people who already had many difficulties in their lives.

One woman spoke of a fire in which she lost all her belongings. She recalled being trapped in her apartment. The World Trade Center attacks brought back this horrible experience in that she identified with the pain of those who were trapped in the buildings. She was so disturbed by these feelings that she had great difficulty sleeping and functioning in her everyday life.

Another individual was directly involved. Steve, a man in his late twenties, was attending classes downtown. He had been suffering from a mental illness since his teens and had come a long way in learning how to live independently and function effectively in society. Luckily, Steve was not in class during the attacks, but his school was closed down for weeks following the disaster. After the school reopened, he had to attend classes in an environment that constantly reminded him of what had happened. The horrible odor that emanated throughout downtown Manhattan penetrated into the classroom, and he also had a clear view of Ground Zero.

Steve was now facing many difficulties. He could not cope with attending classes in a location that reminded him of the disaster, so he finally decided that he needed to drop his hardest class of the semester. He was unable to take care of the simplest tasks anymore. Taking his medications, getting out of bed, food shopping and even just enjoying life became daily obstacles. At the same time, he was experiencing several chronic medical problems that had been exacerbated by the stress following the disaster, including painful leg and kidney problems. Steve was unable to find appropriate medical care, bring himself to take care of his numerous insurance problems, or set up his much-needed appointments. His thought patterns became disrupted as well. Every time he sat down to read, he became paranoid. He thought about future attacks constantly and at one point stopped drinking the water or showering for fear of additional attacks. The media did not make Steve feel any better. With a new threat everyday, he was so terrified, he could not move forward in his chores. To make matters worse, Steve had a close friend with a serious mental illness whom he needed to check on periodically.

Steve was very confused. Would he get his money back for his dropped class? What kind of grade would show up on his transcript? He could not even cope with doing work for the two classes he kept. What would he do if his high-rise building were attacked? How would he get his medication? Would he physically be able to get away with his injured leg? These were all things that Steve thought about constantly and that prevented him from moving along with his life.

Providing counseling services for Steve was a challenge. I had very little experience in counseling, so assisting people following the nation's tragedy seemed impossible. The biggest challenge was to figure out what to do first, considering that this program provided only short-term counseling for a maximum of three sessions. Thankfully, my mental health classes came in handy. In just three sessions, I knew I could make a difference, even if it was small.

After attending the counseling courses, I knew that my plan would be to first determine Steve's most pressing problem. After some discussions, Steve and I decided that getting his medical affairs in order was the most important issue. I advised him to get a notebook and folder in order to organize tasks and information, such as names, bills and phone numbers. He became so overwhelmed even by this, so we worked on breaking each aspect down into small tasks. He also needed to get a calendar to organize his medication schedule, which he had told me that he never seemed to be able to manage.

In the end, I felt as though I made a small difference in focusing Steve to begin his recovery and start the process of getting his life organized again. My studies in occupational therapy helped me to problem solve. Steve and I made a list of all his problems and then prioritized this list in order to help us stay on track. We picked one problem, developed an organizational plan and addressed it. Steve desperately needed resources, information, and referrals to medical and mental health professionals, and this type of practical counseling was able to provide him with this much-needed information. Finally, Steve needed to hear what typical reactions to disasters were, because he thought he was "crazy." Although Steve's life did not change following our sessions, his mind was put at ease, and he felt as though he could start moving forward to put his life back together.

I personally experienced difficulties when providing crisis-counseling services. Allowing periods of silence for Steve to contemplate his thoughts was challenging and I needed to learn that he benefited from this in order to process his feelings. Dealing with Steve's intense reactions was difficult and I found myself getting wrapped up in his emotions. I realized that I was better at dealing with the practical issues than the emotional ones. Steve was facing so many problems and I could not get him to focus on just one. His preexisting physical and mental issues, and decreased access to medical care and mental health counseling were equally significant concerns. Redirecting Steve to remain on just one issue was difficult, as the numerous issues that needed to be addressed were overwhelming us both. Finally, closure was an issue. Although I informed Steve from the beginning that I could help him only over the course of three sessions, he did not understand that this was short-term counseling. I was able to provide him with a referral, but he did not want these sessions to end.

Although my fieldwork ended in November and my crisis counseling sessions came to an end, I did not stop using the techniques I learned through my fieldwork and crisis counseling experiences. My final Fieldwork II placement, which started in January 2002, was at a nursery school located just blocks from Ground Zero. It was only after I started the affiliation that I realized what the teachers and students had faced just four months earlier. The students were in school the day of the tragedy. The teachers reported that during the attack, most students were unaware of what was happening around them. In order to protect the children, the staff sang and danced to divert the children's attention from the people running, the debris falling, and the darkness the falling buildings had brought over the area.

Many of the children had parents who worked at the World Trade Center, and two children sadly lost a parent. Therefore, the children were dealing with a tremendous amount of stress. Most of the students had moved away because of the tragedy and very few students were left at the school. For those who still attended the nursery, they wondered where many of their friends had gone. Even if these families remained in the area, almost all of them needed to relocate because their apartments were destroyed or they had a view of Ground Zero. Moving caused them an additional amount of stress. Others were home at the time and actually witnessed the event.

From the Federal Emergency Management Agency courses, I learned a significant amount of information regarding typical reactions of children to a crisis. Although I was not at this fieldwork placement to deal with the effects that the disaster brought upon the children, I tried to be of assistance when needed. As I developed the trust of the students and their families, I learned more about their individual experiences with the tragedies. One woman said that she was in one of the buildings that collapsed and most of her coworkers were killed. Her daughter was now frightened that she would lose her mother every day when her mother went to work. They had to move, which added to her daughter's trauma.

Another mother, Kim, was just about to move abroad. She came to me right before her move because she knew I was a "therapist." Kim told me that her children were home that day. Her family watched the second plane hit the second building. Kim said that she became hysterical and the family had to escape the building so quickly that they did not even have time to put on their shoes. Kim felt so guilty about the way she had acted and thought that she had a negative impact on her children. She indicated that whenever her three-year-old daughter sees a New York City map, she traces with her fingers the route the planes took to crash into the towers. Kim was terrified now. She was scared about how her children would handle traveling by plane, the relocation of her family to a different country, and most importantly, how the disaster had affected her children. Although I was not able to have a formal session with her, from the crisis counseling experience, I was able to provide her with basic information about normal reactions to this event, coping strategies, and ways that children typically react to experiencing a traumatic event. I was also able to provide her with resources of whom to go to and what to look for in her children should she want to seek out professional help.

Observing the children during their playtime allowed me to see how this tragedy impacted them as well. I often saw children act out their feelings while I was playing with them during free time. One five-year-old boy was building a tower out of blocks. He then crashed it down and without prompts from me, he began to tell me his story about how he had to evacuate his home, take a ferry to New Jersey, and stay at a stranger's home on September eleventh. Although he also seemed frightened, he seemed relieved to share this story and have an opportunity to express his feelings.

Parents reported that their children had started to act out, that they could not sleep, or that they have become very quiet since the incident. As an occupational therapy student, I found that engaging the children in activities gave them a chance to talk about what happened. Additionally, because some children were between two and three years of age and could not yet discuss emotions, this provided them with the chance to act out what was making them sad.

The September eleventh attacks brought many tragedies to New York City. Amongst those who were most affected were children and those with mental and physical disabilities. Although my crisis counseling experience was limited, I sought to help in any way I could. Project Liberty gave me the opportunity to do just that. Through this experience, I witnessed how the nature of human beings to pull together and help one another in times of great distress was so powerful regardless of an individual's age or limitations.

NOTE

1. Names and personal details have been changed to protect the privacy of consumers.

REFERENCES

American Red Cross in Greater New York. (2001). *How do I deal with my feelings?* [Brochure].

Center for Mental Health Services. (2000). *Staff roles and services within crisis counseling programs.* Rockville, MD: Center for Mental Health Services.

DeWolfe, D. J. (2000). *Field manual for mental health and human service workers in major disasters.* Washington, D.C.: National Mental Health Services Knowledge Exchange Network.

Coping with the Trauma of 9/11

Jane Prawda, MA, OTR, MS/Ed

Why some people experience Post-Traumatic Stress Disorder (PTSD) while others do not remains to be seen, but a recent study suggests that inheriting a shorter version of a single gene appears to predispose people to fear. Using magnetic resonance imaging, Dr. Ahmad R. Hariri and Dr. Daniel R. Weinberger, at the National Institute of Mental Health, established a direct link between a genetic variation and the behavior of a region of the brain called the amygdala, which processes fear (Nagourney, 2002). It appears that genetics, when combined with other factors including environment, past experiences in life, age, support system, feelings of safety, a coexisting psychiatric illness, long-term physical illness, and ability to cope with adverse situations, influence the development of PTSD.

This chapter examines the latter, coping mechanisms, through two case examples (Cillis, D.R., personal communication, June, 2002 & Licari, A., personal communication, June, 2002) of people affected by the 9/11 disaster and possible interventions for return to a healthy, productive life.

Dr. Daniel R. Cillis, a professor and former military officer, was on jury duty and found himself in the vicinity of the World Trade Center at the time of the disaster. The following is a transcript of a personal diary entry he made on September 11, 2001.

A Day to Remember. I was downtown today. As I got off at the Wall Street subway station thousands of people were looking up at

---

[Haworth co-indexing entry note]: "Coping with the Trauma of 9/11." Prawda, Jane. Co-published simultaneously in *Occupational Therapy in Mental Health* (The Haworth Press, Inc.) Vol. 19, No. 3/4, 2003, pp. 145-151; and: *Surviving 9/11: Impact and Experiences of Occupational Therapy Practitioners* (ed: Pat Precin) The Haworth Press, Inc., 2003, pp. 145-151. Single or multiple copies of this article are available for a fee from The Haworth Document Delivery Service [1-800-HAWORTH, 9:00 a.m. - 5:00 p.m. (EST). E-mail address: docdelivery@haworthpress.com].

Digital Object Identifier: 10.1300/J004v19n03_13

145

the fire in both towers. It was amazing. Then, all hell broke loose as the first building came down. We all ran like mad away from the horrible dust and fragments. As we ran away from one black cloud of death, ANOTHER came at us from the other end of the street. It seemed like certain death, but with seconds before the two clouds hit I jumped into a building. I was trapped there for an hour. The streets looked like a nuclear winter. Everything was covered with gray dust six inches thick and it was dark. The deadly missiles were laying everywhere. The building filled with smoke so I decided not to die like a rat and ran out toward the river where there was a minimum of breathable air. Then it took 4 hours to walk home. . . . I will never forget this day.

Dr. Cillis later remarked that he was in a state of high alert while trapped in the building. He reported, "I made a decision *not* to stay in the building [but to] take my chances [and] head for the river. This was tantamount to controlling my environment." Dr. Cillis stated that the leadership from Mayor Rudolph Giuliani gave him hope. He recalls the Mayor proclaiming, "We are going to overcome it."

Daniel describes his impressions of what it was like in New York City twelve days later in an e-mail he sent to his friend Ron Licari in New Mexico. The following are excerpts:

Ron: To be in New York these days is to bear witness to staggering heroism. We will never forget it. The anxiety is overwhelming at times. People are not sleeping wondering what is next. Everything has changed, perhaps forever . . . Day by day, inch by inch the city is getting better. The lights went back on around the World Trade Center for residents who live close. Over 12,000 were blacked out by the attack. Baseball came back and the Mets are amazing! They have not lost since the attack and are closing in on the Braves and Phillies. Of course, the Yankees are already in the playoffs . . . DC [Daniel Cillis].

On the three-month anniversary of 9/11, Dr. Cillis returned to Ground Zero. Returning to the site helped him "enter the recovery stage," he stated. However, eleven months after the World Trade Center disaster he shuts down when questioned about what he had experienced.

Dr. Cillis utilized various coping mechanisms at different stages of his healing from the disaster. The first was controlling his environment demonstrated by his willful escape out of a smoke-filled building to the water where the air was cleaner. Once home, he wrote journal entries in a diary and utilized his social network to e-mail his friends about his experiences and what had transpired. He then was able to experience hope through the words of an authority figure, the Mayor. And finally, he used in vivo exposure when he visited Ground Zero three months after 9/11.

The literature supports the effectiveness of Dr. Cillis's coping strategies. Dr. Viktor Frankl, a German psychiatrist and Holocaust survivor, has written extensively about being able to control one's environment. He comments about how he coped with the Holocaust by finding comfort in realizing that he alone controls his thoughts, memories and reactions (Frankl, 2000). It is thought that people who lack social supports are more likely to develop PTSD than those who have and utilize strong social networks (Yehuda et al., 1998). Bessel A. van der Kolk, MD (Korn, medscape 408691, 2002), researcher in the area of psychiatry, PTSD and related phenomena, warns that people who shut down are also at risk for PTSD. In vivo exposure or exposure therapy promotes confrontation with feared objects, situations, memories, and images. In Dr. Cillis's case, it involved a visit to the place where he was trapped. According to Rothbaum and Schwartz (2002), noted researchers in the field of PTSD, the most effective method for treating PTSD is exposure therapy. Exposure therapy can include exposing a person to the traumatic event through imaging, in vivo, and/or virtual reality, and includes such techniques as flooding and systematic desensitization.

Other methods proven effective in desensitizing trauma include stress inoculation training, cognitive behavioral therapy, and eye movement desensitization and reprocessing (EMDR). Stress inoculation training uses relaxation, thought stopping, and cognitive restructuring techniques. Dr. Joseph LeDoux (Goleman, 1995, p. 213), a neuroscientist, conjectures, "Once your emotional system learns something, it seems you never let it go. What therapy does is teaches your neurocortex how to inhibit your amygdala. The propensity to act is suppressed, while your basic emotion remains but in a subdued form." EMDR begins with the client imagining the upsetting trauma. When the client's emotions become overwhelming and the client begins to sob (the client's frontal lobes have now shut down and the limbic system has taken over as shown on MRI), the healer says, "Stay there, feel that in your body" (Korn, medscape 408691, 2002). Immediately following this, the client exhibits bilateral eye movements and the intensity of the emotion decreases (Korn, medscape 408691, 2002). EMDR is effective with clients who are too upset to speak because it decreases stress by using feelings instead of verbal descriptions.

Children are very vulnerable and can be easily traumatized by an event such as 9/11, including those who have viewed the destruction of the Towers over and over again on television. Yael Danieli, PhD, (Korn, medscape 408692, 2002) clinician and trauma specialist, affirms, "Children did not have to look at it over and over again to experience the trauma. Everybody talked about it anyhow."

Ariel Licari, from Rio Rancho, New Mexico, turned 13 years old on September 11, 2001. She appeared to have no symptoms of anxiety related to 9/11. She stated that the disaster seemed "unreal. . . . Actually, it felt like a nightmare." Ariel said in a strong voice, "We are going to win over terrorism." When questioned, she agreed that her parents and teachers helped her manage her feelings as did writing the following report about 9/11 that she presented to her class the same day.

Terror in the United States

Today is September 11th of 2001. Today an airplane crashed into one of the most important buildings in the United States, the World Trade Center. I watched the news in the morning at 7:00 a.m. I heard that there was a plane crash so I was interested in watching. I was interested because I like to see what is going on around me. What was going on was that a plane was hijacked and purposely was crashed into the WTC. Then ten minutes later a second plane hit the tower. When I was watching the news it was just after the first plane hit and the news station was taking calls from eyewitnesses. A girl called in and she saw the whole thing and while she was talking the second plane hit the other tower. Later when I was at school, I went to my first elective when we talked more deeply about it. We then heard that the Pentagon building in the US Capital had also been hit. They evacuated the White House and there was and still is a whole bunch of chaos.

After lunch, I went to science and we did our assignment and when we were finished we turned on the TV and we saw things we already saw on the TV before and then we saw the people from another country cheering. They were cheering because the United States was getting attacked; I mean they were literally happy.

When I got home my dad was worried about his friend, Dan (Dr. Dan Cillis) because Dan lives in Manhattan, New York. We talked about this whole thing as a family and my sister, Melissa, who is eight didn't seem to know what was going on. Later, my dad got ahold of a friend that got a call from Dan–he was all right.

I hope the people whose families live in New York are doing all right. I hope that other people don't die. I think that it is wrong to do this kind of thing to other countries, but the other countries do not think that way. I think that it feels like a dream, a really realistic nightmare. I pray for those who have been affected.

Dr. Danieli (Korn, medscape 408692, 2002) comments further on how children were affected by 9/11:

> We have lots and lots of children in the city and around the country watching [television]. We have a lot of adults being very anxious and feeling vulnerable. And they are the parents and the teachers and they are those whose function is to protect, be all-powerful, and containing like a protective membrane against the evil of the world. That has been shaken. . . . A lot of children are terrified. In a funny way, some of them are much more openly articulate about their feelings than are the adults.

To help children cope, the protective and containing function of the family must be reinstated. One way to do this is for the whole family to establish a new normality where children participate in purposeful activities and a bereavement process. Encouraging children to talk more about the rescuers and the helpful deeds that were done may help them develop a more balanced view of good and evil in relation to the disaster. Participating in activities that are helpful to the cause can help children feel a part of the situation instead of feeling helpless.

In the aftermath of the disaster, even though time has created some psychological distance, images remain embedded in our minds. Why has 9/11 had such a profound effect on our national psyche? Harriet Braiker, PhD, clinical psychologist, replies, "In part it is because we can no longer tell ourselves with assuredness that we are safe, or that our children or parents are safe; we can only hope, pray, and try to avoid danger even though we cannot know if, when or where it may come from next" (Braiker, 2002, p. 17).

Dr. Braiker identifies "The September 11 Syndrome."

> Those people affected by the disaster that had no direct connection with the disaster produced symptoms of a collective acute stress reaction across America. The impact obviously was greater if you

were near Ground Zero or other attack sites, but make no mistake: the collective acute stress reaction I am describing was, and is, a national phenomenon. (Braiker, 2002, p. 4)

Dr. Braiker describes seven steps to healing (Braiker, 2002, p. 63):

1. Controlling the Images in Your Mind
2. Controlling Negative Thoughts
3. Overcoming Specific Fears and Anxieties
4. Overcoming Helplessness and Depression
5. Creating a Comfort Zone
6. Making Connections
7. Finding Personal Courage

Responses to the trauma of 9/11 are unique in many ways, ranging from acute stress to PTSD. Adaptive and maladaptive responses include: adaptive denial, returning to powerful feelings of connection with other people, feeling of control over the environment, "fight or flight" response, depression, numbing, alcohol and/or substance abuse, increased arousal or hypervigilance, avoidance, shock, horror, feelings related to symbols of patriotism, functional impairment, significant stress, negative thinking, turning to government leadership for symbols of hope, anxiety, fear, hopelessness, helplessness, vulnerability, and grieving. Coping styles are indicative of personal needs. Treatment includes: exposure or in vivo therapy, stress-inoculation training, cognitive behavior therapy, EMDR, social support groups, and bereavement and grief counseling. The occupational therapist can take an active role in the assessment and treatment of PTSD and related disorders. The emotional state of Americans of all ages in the aftermath of 9/11 will need to be assessed for years to come.

REFERENCES

Braiker, H. B. (2002). *The September 11 syndrome.* New York: McGraw-Hill, pp. 4, 17, 63, 64-151.

Frankl, V. (2000). *Man's search for meaning.* Boston: Beacon Press.

Goleman, D. (1995). *Emotional intelligence.* New York: Random House, p. 213.

Korn, M. L. (2002). *Trauma and PTSD: Aftermaths of the WTC disaster–An interview with Bessel A. van der Kolk, MD.* Medscape. Retrieved June, 2002 from *www.medscape.com/viewarticle/408691*

Korn, M. L. (2002). *Trauma and PTSD: Aftermaths of the WTC disaster–An interview with Yael Danieli, PhD.* Medscape. Retrieved June, 2002 from *www.medscape.com/viewarticle/408692*

Nagourney, E. (2002). "Fearing more than fear itself." *New York Times,* July 30, Section F, p.6.

Rothbaum, B. O. & Schwartz, A.C. (2002). Exposure therapy for posttraumatic stress disorder. *American Journal of Psychotherapy; 56,* 59-75.

Yehuda, R., Schmeidler, J., Wainberg, M., Binder-Byrnes, K., & Duvdevani, T. (1998). Vulnerability to posttraumatic stress disorder in adult offspring of Holocaust survivors. *American Journal of Psychiatry; 155,* 1163-1171.

Spiritual Spontaneity:
Developing Our Own 9/11:
One Occupational Therapist's
Spiritual Journey Across the 9/11 Divide

Naomi Schubin Greenberg

The events of 9/11 brought a new awakening to spirituality both within and outside the occupational therapy community. What does 9/11 represent? In the USA, 9/11 clearly marks the events of September 11, 2001 with massive loss of life at three separate sites. Some link the date with the emergency telephone number 911. Outside of the USA the date is not as significant as the term "Twin Towers" referring to Manhattan's World Trade Center with the focus on the symbols and the greater loss of life in New York City than at the other sites in Pennsylva-

---

[Haworth co-indexing entry note]: "Spiritual Spontaneity: Developing Our Own 9/11: One Occupational Therapist's Spiritual Journey Across the 9/11 Divide." Greenberg, Naomi Schubin. Co-published simultaneously in *Occupational Therapy in Mental Health* (The Haworth Press, Inc.) Vol. 19, No. 3/4, 2003, pp. 153-189; and: *Surviving 9/11: Impact and Experiences of Occupational Therapy Practitioners* (ed: Pat Precin) The Haworth Press, Inc., 2003, pp. 153-189. Single or multiple copies of this article are available for a fee from The Haworth Document Delivery Service [1-800-HAWORTH, 9:00 a.m. - 5:00 p.m. (EST). E-mail address: docdelivery@haworthpress.com].

http://www.haworthpress.com/web/OTMH
Digital Object Identifier: 10.1300/J004v19n03_14

153

nia and Washington, DC. The sites have been called hallowed ground, a reference to a spiritual connection.

Tom Otterness's *Nine-Eleven* response (Photo 1) focuses on New York City using the figures of sculptures he had previously created. Inspirational works touch the emotions. *Nine-Eleven* is clearly moving. "Rendered in tones of red, the watercolor depicts the figure of *Gulliver* reclining on the island of Manhattan, his body extending from the Brooklyn Bridge to the George Washington Bridge. Across the Hudson River in New Jersey sits the figure of *Crying Giant*, the grief-filled observer" (Tsai, 2002, p. 4). Otterness based *Gulliver* on the classic story *Gulliver's Travels*, in which the giant is captured by little people. Does the shackled *Gulliver* in *Nine-Eleven* show innocent bewilderment or is he sadly recognizing his predicament? Could this be an example of spiritual humility? In the two lonely figures can we also sense tears, helplessness, a feeling of abandonment and despair? Post-9/11 reports implied that any one of these could be a catalyst for looking heavenward for hope or a plea for turning their plight over to a power greater than us. And do we the observers sense the urge to reach out to these people in need? That too, is spiritual. Researcher Barbara Fredrickson's post-9/11 research found that those who reach out to one another are more resilient than other people (Michaud, 2002).

I saw Otterness's *Nine-Eleven* at the Nassau County Art Museum where his whimsical sculptures, which have included *Lighten Up: Art with a Sense of Humor* (2001), provide a great contrast. I found myself connecting personally with the rivers in *Nine-Eleven*. I was born in Hoboken, New Jersey, not far from where *Crying Giant* sits, worked on Roosevelt Island, depicted in the painting, and now teach in Long Island City across the East River from *Gulliver*. LaGuardia Community College still includes watercolor and ceramics as required techniques in its Introduction to Occupational Therapy laboratory course. The *Nine-Eleven* watercolor reminded me of the important therapeutic value of expressing feelings and reflections through art and music. The Public Radio Station, WNYC, released a six-minute CD just after 9/11 that sets an original prayer to Bach's funerary music and ends abruptly as did the ability to broadcast as the World Trade Center buildings tumbled.

We can learn much from our own reflections and those of others as we consider how best to utilize spirituality in the clinical and educational setting. The theory of Spiritual Spontaneity, our own 9/11, is proposed to train or enable us to be ready to face future unanticipated events from a spiritual perspective. The word spiritual has 9 letters, and the word spontaneity has 11. Together they provide a way to use the

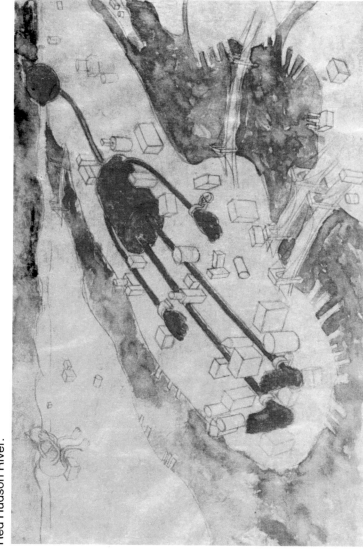

PHOTO 1. *Nine-Eleven*, Watercolor Showing *Gulliver's* Body Shackled and Stretched Across the Island of Manhattan While the *Crying Giant* Sits Filled with Grief on the New Jersey Side of a Blood Red Hudson River.

Water color and pencil on paper by Tom Otterness, 2001. Photo by Dean Brown. Used by permission.

numbers 9-11 for a goal-directed path. The environment has changed. Can we change as well (Greenberg & Heltzel, 2002)? Gandhi said, "Be the change you wish to see in the world" (Weiss & Cecala, 2002).

Little did I know when I submitted my proposal for a spirituality presentation (Greenberg, 2001) at the New York State Occupational Therapy Association (NYSOTA) Annual Conference that the topic would take on a whole new meaning. Just two months after 9/11, a session on spirituality was, of course, well attended by participants with 9/11 on their minds. The interactive workshop format allowed opportunities for sharing with a focus on healing, reflection and perspective. Several occupational therapy practitioners told how they as New Yorkers had helped their clients and themselves to deal with the aftermath of the World Trade Center crisis. Others shared advice for facing the future. Did both groups already have spiritual spontaneity? Participants were asked the following questions and to share spiritual wisdom for an unpredictable world: What does spiritual or spirituality mean to you? In what way do you or could you use spirituality in your occupational therapy practice? In what ways can spirituality be linked with occupation and/or activity?

The positive spontaneity in Table 1 is mine. That is how the session was handled. I had planned for interaction, an important element in dealing with feelings. One workshop activity was similar to one I had successfully led in Jinotepe, Nicaragua, for special education teachers and United States-based occupational therapy and occupational therapy assistant students. It involved first having participants choose from an array of objects. I had searched in advance through my woodlands, my collection of trinkets from my travels, and my jewelry box for items that could be seen as spiritual. The choices ranged from spruce cones to a yellow wooden sun pin from Jamaica. Some individuals chose to use something they were wearing with which they already had a spiritual linkage. The concept of a circle is unifying, as each person is equidistant from the center. As participants sat in a circle each person shared the reason for choosing the object and a personal spiritual story triggered by

TABLE 1. Words Spontaneously Chosen by Occupational Therapy Practitioners as Representing Spirituality

Belief	Caring	Connection
Faith	Force of life	Hope
Love	Positive spontaneity	Respect
Serenity	Tranquillity	Unity

it. Many chose to connect the item to reflections about 9/11 or to a cultural experience. Post-conference evaluations highlighted the "group interaction exercises" as particularly helpful and asked for more in the future. One therapist's written characterization is perhaps most significant: "A community of souls."

A circle approach is also used by Rachel Naomi Remen (2001), a physician now specializing in counseling individuals with cancer in facilitating workshops for physicians who need to regain their compassion after medical school. She tells of asking physicians to bring an object from home to the workshop and of how she saw a dramatic change in one individual between two workshops. The change was triggered by a stuffed rabbit. Although he had planned only to describe how he had used the stuffed animal to distract young patients, deep meaningful recollections of his youth emerged as he sat in the center.

In a similar vein, while perusing the varied items that had been placed on display just outside Ground Zero, I was reminded, by the cascade of origami cranes among the mementos near Ground Zero (Photo 2), of their spiritual value as described in Remen's *My Grandfather's Blessings* (2000). A surgeon of Japanese heritage made large white paper cranes, the symbol of long life, for many of his patients in advance of their surgery thus "Strengthening Life," the name of the chapter.

Likewise, in *Kitchen Table Wisdom*, Rachel Remen (1997) tells of having created her own unique ring, a face with long hair wrapping around the wearer's finger. She wore it for the first time to a California workshop, was convinced to leave it at the Monterey Peninsula for casting so that others could benefit from its uniqueness, and subsequently learned that it had been washed away in a storm. The title of the chapter is "New Beginnings." In order to begin anew, there first has to be a loss. Is the story representative of an occupation and outlook of a spiritual person? Had Rachel Remen already developed Spiritual Spontaneity through her own experiences with Crohn's disease?

Where did my choice to see situations from a spiritual perspective begin? Appreciation must go first to my parents, William and Edith (Pencak) Schubin, my ultimate role models. I was fortunate in having them into their 90s. Of course, I had lapses in adolescence and beyond. But I can now still draw on their lessons of Spiritual Spontaneity. After a quickly arranged flight from New York to Florida to see my mother in the intensive care unit, almost the first thing she said when she saw me was, "Isn't that a beautiful color?" I first wondered whether the devastating description of her that I had received when the physician called from the emergency room to ask whether I wanted my mother treated

PHOTO 2. A Cascade of Origami: Swans, the Spiritual Significance of Which Is Described by Rachel Naomi Remen, MD, in Her Books.

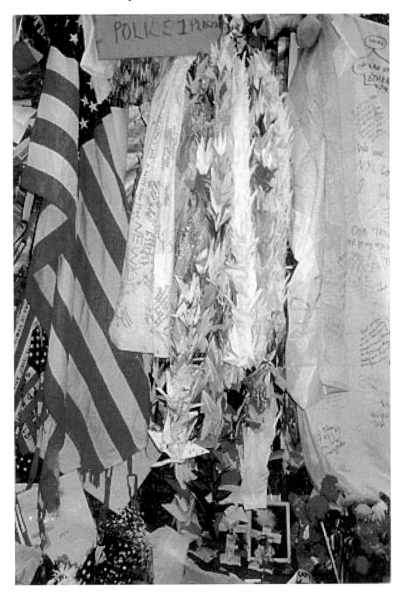

Photo by Naomi Greenberg. Used by permission.

might be accurate. But then she pointed; and I looked; and the color was beautiful! I can still see it now, a wonderful coral mixture of the colors of urine and blood hanging in a see-through bag from her intravenous (IV) pole.

When I stayed in my father's room the night before his surgery during a seven-week turbulent hospital stay, he awoke. Probably thinking I was my mother (their marriage lasted 63 years) he said, "We hope for the best, but if not, let's not be greedy. Not everyone is granted 94 good years." This from a person who had seen his buddies killed in devastating battles in World War I, who had lost almost his entire family in the Holocaust, who had been given only months to live by physicians at Johns Hopkins Hospital forty years previously, who had seen his business destroyed in a fire, and who was now facing what would turn out to be a colostomy. Helen Keller, who achieved fame despite the fact that she was both blind and deaf, said, "Resolve to keep happy, and your joy and you shall form an invincible host against difficulties" (Quotes Happiness 019.0).

We can find case studies of Spiritual Spontaneity in our personal lives and in our professional encounters. When I was doing coverage at a Veteran's Administration facility, I was told to expect that the first patient on my list would not come down to occupational therapy and that someone else could just verify that. I refused the offer and went up to his room myself. Drawing on therapeutic use of self, years of experience, the opportunity to welcome a challenge and my own Spiritual Spontaneity, I briefly established rapport and asked him to do me a favor. "Come down. If you don't like it, I'll take you back." He agreed. At the end of the 45-minute session, he said, "You know, I really enjoyed being here." What made the difference? In that entire room of patients and therapists, he and I were the only ones truly communicating. I had pushed the right buttons. Realizing what the word "veteran" means, I could enable him to share those experiences. He chose to talk about crossing religious lines in relationships with buddies and how these relationships had sustained him in action. Our interaction was the motivation for him to carry out the designated activities toward his physical goals. The others in the room looked and listened in awe. I felt elated in my connection with him and its achievement and sad that with the cost-cutting efficiency of managed care there appear to be fewer opportunities for in-depth interactions in occupational therapy between patient and therapist.

With occupational therapy's increased focus on the use of technology, there is perhaps correspondingly less emphasis on the importance of therapeutic use of self. After September 11th, 2001 our technological society may not be viewed the same way. A high-tech terrorist attack was used on a high-tech society. "There was a sense that this could be a turning point like no other, that perhaps technology will never be viewed in quite the same way," said Robert C. Post, a senior fellow at the Dibner Institute for the History of Science and Religion, in a *New York Times* article (Lohr, 2001, p. 4).

Have we now become a more spiritual nation? What does the aftermath of September 11, 2001 mean spiritually for occupational therapy practitioners and the recipients of occupational therapy services? Should spirituality content be included in packets the American Occupational Therapy Foundation is considering for dealing with the impact? Could spirituality become an emerging area of practice? Is a Special Interest Section on spirituality on the horizon for the future? Spiritual Spontaneity can be taught, can be evaluated and can be developed as a preventative and therapeutic measure.

In the post-9/11 session of a spiritual disciplines stress management group I have been leading for ten years, the mental/spiritual imagery finally enabled participants to experience a transition from negative energy to positive potential. Individuals were asked, with their eyes closed, to picture themselves on a soft comfortable cloud floating slowly past ground zero and onward to a place of serenity (perhaps a nature spot) where they had felt positive inspiration in the past. In similar ways individuals and groups can be trained to spontaneously move into spiritual imagery in relation to a stressful event. In Associated Press photographer Mark Phillips' photograph of the smoke rising from the World Trade Center tower, "Many say they can see eyes, a nose, a mouth" (Wells & Maher, 2001). With imagination, it is a face, and it takes imagination to move us beyond the immediate reality to the potential of what can be. It was Albert Einstein, the century's most famous scientist, who said, "Imagination is more important than knowledge" (Viereck, 1929).

Psychologist Miriam Adahan, who developed her spiritual disciplines model based on Recovery Inc. Organization's four-step example (Low, 1997), discusses the remarkable ability of the mind to change. A key aspect is to focus on the concept that we have choices, that we can choose a spiritual response. "The ability to consciously maximize or minimize the importance of events in your life is a skill which can be developed and honed through constant exercise" (Adahan, 1995, p. 230).

I am reminded of a full-day workshop on brain research that I attended. One of the areas emphasized was that of the lazy brain. "Just try changing your silverware drawer." How many of us are on automatic pilot in our responses? Is it habit that has us following the masses even in the way we think about events? If we truly want to develop our ability to see events from a spiritual perspective, we may have to retrain ourselves to do so.

Recognizing the importance to both patient and health care provider, medical schools are increasingly offering spirituality courses. Stimulated by ethical principles and patient-centered care, ninety medical schools were offering such courses in 2002. The introduction of a new full course on spirituality to the curriculum of an occupational therapy program (The Sage Colleges) was announced at the NYSOTA spirituality session. Some ask, what can be taught to fill a full course? *Faith, Spirituality and Medicine* (King, 2000) includes research linking religious practices and health, a biopsychosocial-spiritual model, health beliefs of selected religious groups, mobilizing spiritual resources, taking a spiritual history, clinical experience, ethics and more. Perhaps another topic is Spiritual Spontaneity.

In "The Spirit of Medicine," Christina Puchalsky (2002, p. 6), Founder and Director of the George Washington Institute for Spirituality and Medicine, states that, "The courses emphasize that health-care providers address their own inner sources of strength, their spiritual beliefs and whatever gives them meaning in their professional lives and helps them cope with the stresses. . . . I want to talk about how people come to understand meaning and purpose in their lives and how they cope with suffering." The death of almost 3,000 persons on 9/11/2001 reminds us that the time of loss is unpredictable. Therefore, we can try to prepare by developing a special coping skill, Spiritual Spontaneity.

Psychiatrist Keith Meador (2002, p. 7), Director of the Duke University Institute on Care at the End of Life, the first of its kind in the nation, states, "Most of us assume we will live forever. We think, 'I won't die; it's other people who do that.'" "Making Peace with Fear" (Graham, 2002, p. 58) gives a similar message with role models but goes on to say, "Letting go into life may not be easy, but it's the one sure pathway to wisdom and joy."

After being thanked profusely while visiting the home of a family in mourning that had lost a brother and fiancé in the disaster, I decided to join another family for a memorial service at Ground Zero. Neither family had had a body recovered. Ten weeks after the tragedy, I accompanied the sister, the parents and others on two chartered buses. It was awesome as we came out into the opening after following a narrow path, to see the one remaining recognizable remnant of the façade of the

World Trade Center standing alone like a steeple pointed toward the heavens (Photo 3). While the group recited psalms on a special memorial platform, an arc of water sprayed the still smoldering tower (Photo 4). Individuals viewed the small flags that represented the countries of victims of the attack painted on the back wall of the platform (Photo 5). An array of emergency vehicles stood by while a battering ram hanging from a crane slowly worked to demolish a building with the hope of still finding human remains (Photo 6). As we were told that another group was waiting to memorialize its dead, I reflected on what made the experience so moving. Perhaps it was the group collectiveness–that we could be there for one another; perhaps it was the sense of purpose; perhaps it was the key recognition that life has meaning. Or was it the words of the firefighter who led us to the platform with instructions, "It's okay to cry. We've all been there."

Similar words were expressed in *Oprah Magazine* by N. Hirschfeld (2002, p. 22) who started a voluntary support group for fellow police officers and teaches, "It's okay to cry. It's okay to hurt." She reexamined her grief and focused on newfound values asking, "What in God's name are we meant to do with the rest of our lives?" We are asked to trust both the joy and the pain of our lives as part of our sense of purpose. We need to absorb unexpected situations and be changed by them toward new or modified goals. A talent for serendipity is helpful: the ability to convert what others consider accidents or misfortunes into something useful. As in the *Paradoxical Commandments*, "The good you do today may be forgotten tomorrow; do good anyway!" (Keith, 2002).

It is this ability to see smaller and larger events, even a 9/11, from a particular perspective that may be considered spiritual. What is Spiritual Spontaneity? The *Oxford English Dictionary* identifies the derivation of "spirituality" from Latin and French. *Spiration* and *spirare* refer to breath and breathing. Some identify this as the breath transferred to the first human being, which makes humans different from other living things such as plants and animals. Thus, individuals are able to develop Spiritual Spontaneity. Inspiration refers to both a phase of breathing and to an experience or thought that can promote awareness or move us in new directions. We can work with the breath, the life spiral. The *Merriam-Webster Dictionary* defines "spontaneous" as "produced freely, done naturally." Synonyms include "instinctive" and "automatic." Spiritual spontaneity can then be considered a readiness to respond spiritually to the unexpected.

What does Spiritual Spontaneity have to do with 9/11? Although 9/11 was a shock like no other, the media and the Office of Homeland Security are warning us to expect the unexpected. Some people respond

PHOTO 3. The One Remaining Recognizable Remnant of the Façade of the World Trade Center.

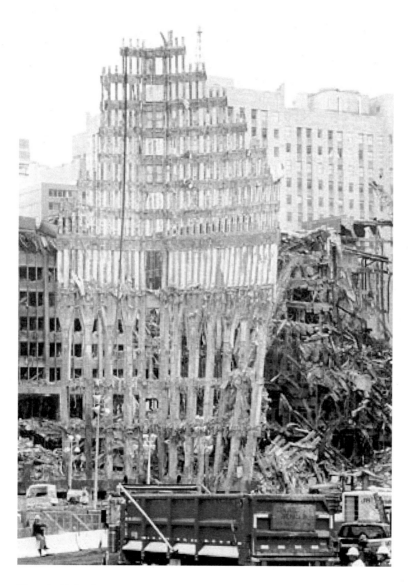

Photo by Helen Rosenstark. Used by permission.

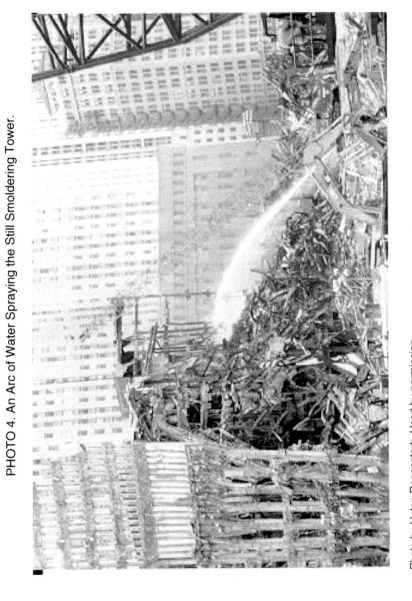

PHOTO 4. An Arc of Water Spraying the Still Smoldering Tower.

Photo by Helen Rosenstark. Used by permission.

PHOTO 5. Individual Viewing Flags Representing Countries of the Victims of the Attack Painted on the Back Wall of a Platform.

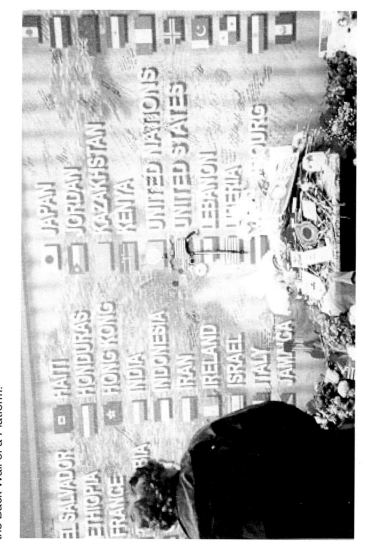

PHOTO 6. Emergency Vehicles Stand by While a Battering Ram Suspended from a Crane Works Slowly to Demolish a Building in Hopes of Still Finding Human Remains.

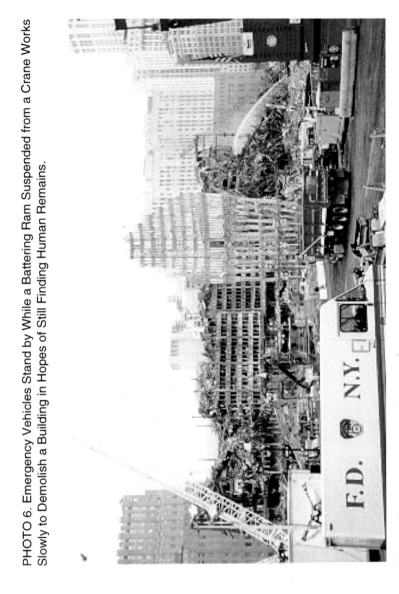

Photo by Helen Rosenstark. Used by permission.

by not venturing into crowds, the subway, bridges or whatever else is suggested as a potential target at the moment. Others stew in worry or share their concerns wherever they may be. The rest of us, if motivated, can develop our Spiritual Spontaneity and motivate our clients to do so as well. One of the measures of mental health is how quickly a person can recoup after a setback or upsetting situation. One of the measures of Spiritual Spontaneity is how quickly a person can find a spiritual perspective after an unanticipated event or disaster. Both an occupational therapy article (Cotrell, 2001) and a *Prevention* magazine article use the term "resilience" and highlight its importance. Both include references to 9/11 with the latter offering a test of resilience (Michaud, 2002).

Just three weeks after 9/11, I was having a medical check-up. The physician, considering expectations of stress factors, asked me about my reaction to 9/11. I was able to answer with what I considered to be an immediate spiritual response by describing the following: A psychologist colleague told me of having experienced three incidents of being near terrorist attacks in another country, and remarked "I don't believe in fate (faith), but . . . " When I mentioned it to my son in the same country, his reaction was, "What does it take to wake someone up?" Is such a remark an example of conditioning? Or is it commitment? Franklin D. Roosevelt, the USA president who used a wheelchair said, "Physical force can never permanently withstand the impact of spiritual force" (Band of Angels and Bits and Pieces).

The August 7, 2002 edition of the *Journal of the American Medical Association (JAMA)* featured both a research article and an editorial article related to the increase in post-traumatic stress syndrome (PTSD) following 9/11. Reports of the mental health impact have also noted a significantly greater impact on New Yorkers than the rest of the country (North, 2002, and Schlenger et al., 2002). A follow-up report gave the statistic of 1 in 10 New Yorkers with PTSD. Yet, *JAMA* raised questions about the diagnosis, as the *Diagnostic and Statistical Manual IV (DSM IV)* (American Psychiatric Association, 2000) does not identify television viewing as one of the qualifying events. Post-trauma research could be done successfully following 9/11 because research populations were already identified for other purposes.

September eleventh presented us with examples of family life and ways of coping with loss. Many people anxiously followed the daily biographies of those lost in the World Trade Center. A compilation in *Portraits: 9/11/01* (Emerson, 2002) is featured in conjunction with the *Yahrtzeit* (anniversary of death) exhibit at the Museum of the Jewish Heritage, just south of Ground Zero. In "Dealing with the Loss of a

Loved One Through Celebration" (Swanson, 2002), recent research on the topic of grieving and spirituality is cited as confirming that prayer helps. The article indicates that "those left behind are in a continual state of reinvesting in the relationship. Memorials and services held to honor the dead keep that investment alive and well" (Swanson, 2002, p. 24). All new plans for Ground Zero include a memorial park. During an August 2002 visit to Ground Zero, I noted that the firefighters' memorial at the Hudson River, just west of the site, has a plaque with the phrase from the pledge of allegiance, "One nation under God."

Spirituality is drawing increasing attention in occupational therapy as in other helping professions. The *American Journal of Occupational Therapy* devoted a full issue to the subject in 1997. A more recent article concluded that there were diverse views of spirituality among therapists (Taylor, 2000). There was no consensus as to its meaning. Mark Rosenfeld discusses how spirituality can be used as a therapeutic approach, referring to occupational performance and the use of prayer groups in occupational therapy (Rosenfeld, 2000). Holiday traditions have been cited as useful to achieve therapeutic goals (Greenberg & Lewis, 1995). Table 2 gives examples of potential spiritual activities. A proposal to specifically add spirituality as an area of assessment was rejected in 2002 by the American Occupational Therapy Association because the topic is included in *Occupational Therapy Practice Framework Domain and Process*. Spiritual is identified as a context and defined as "the fundamental orientation of a person's life; that which inspires and motivates that individual" (AOTA, 2002, p. 63). Jacobs defines spiritual as the "nonphysical and nonmaterial aspect of existence, which contributes insight into the nature and meaning of a person's life" (2001, p. 180). Steinsaltz contrasts the physical world with the spiritual world. "The spiritual world is, first and foremost, all the things we relate to through our minds. This includes our thoughts and emotions, love, hate,

TABLE 2. Potential Spiritual Activities for Therapeutic Use

Book of reflections	Inspirational book discussion
Construction of traditional objects	Learning group
Crane origami	Poetry therapy
Creative prayer project	Reminiscence group
Cultural diversity sharing	Spiritual imaginary relaxation exercise
Genogram with spiritual occupations	Spiritual object circle
Hands-on project	Therapeutic adaptation of ritual items

and envy, the ability to read, to enjoy music, or to solve equations, to know that we exist, and to relate to others" (Steinsaltz, 2001, pp. 54-55).

What was it that triggered my recent professional spiritual renaissance? Clearly, the spirituality workshop at the World Federation of Occupational Therapists Congress in Montreal was a highlight. Instead of individual presentations from England, Alabama and Scotland (Hume, 1998, Mayers, 1998, & Thibodaux, 1998), an open forum was held. The unexpectedly large turnout was an endorsement for recognition of the place for spirituality within occupational therapy. In a huge room the give and take featured perspectives from places as diverse as Hong Kong and Wales. An occupational therapy student from McGill University told how, using meditation and breathing, she was able to integrate Eastern concepts of spirituality with Western views as a result of her parents' origins from very different backgrounds: "We need to have an understanding of silence." An educator from the University of Toronto described the college's two-day overnight workshops in a quiet setting using verbal and non-verbal images and thoughts about spirituality. Perhaps in anticipation of a potential 9/11, another participant suggested creating hope banks: "Trauma often brings people to spirituality. . . . Spirituality might be used to develop hope."

Stimulated by that session, I encouraged occupational therapy assistant students at LaGuardia Community College to create a booklet entitled *Cultural Diversity in Spirituality* (Greenberg & Lewis, 1995). Students shared their own personal experiences and perspectives and interviewed other members of the college community. Entries representing more than thirty countries, cultures or religions show why Queens County in New York City is considered one of the most diverse in the USA. Following are some comments by occupational therapy assistant students with their chosen identity: Trinidad: "Despite all that goes on, one is only as sick as the soul and mind are." Puerto Rican heritage (a legally blind artist): "By looking at what is beautiful in nature, I was inspired to recreate beauty in objects, just as God (the creator) has done. This is very spiritual to me because it brings my mind and body to a place where I forget myself and focus on the feeling of uninhibited doing." Punjabi, India: "Spirituality is the connection energy of individual and life. During the cultural dance, Bhangara, individuals throw hands up in the air to celebrate increased energy and spirituality as a group." Hindu: "Eating meat is prohibited because it makes you angry by nature while yoga touches the spiritual senses." Ireland: "Spirituality teaches medical staff to be humane. I was brought up in a society that has deep traditions and spiritual beliefs including use of a secret potion of herbs."

Jamaica: "The sect Kumina uses drumbeaters who sit in a circle as they try to make contact with the dead." Bolivia: "Among the Guarini Indians, the oldest man in the tribe burns some herbs believing that the spirits will come from the sky and cure the sick person. In most cases, the person gets better." Bangladesh: "I was born into a Muslim family. Believing in the Supreme Being keeps you from feeling hopeless. It does not matter what religion you follow; if you follow it properly, it makes you a better human being."

In introducing the LaGuardia booklet, I wrote, "Walking the boardwalk, the sensations that brought a smile to my face, joy to my heart, and a sense of contentment to my mind included seeing the beam of moonlight on the water, hearing a little frog jumping out of the grass, smelling and almost tasting the sea air, and touching the cool fine sand." On a boardwalk just about 18 miles from Ground Zero, I was again able to capture that same inspiration post- 9/11. An Educational Development grant allowed me to design an inspirational book project in conjunction with a mental health occupational therapy laboratory class focusing on group process. Each student was to select a book found inspirational, to share highlights with the class, to connect some of the ideas with occupational therapy and to prepare a brief summary for an annotated bibliography. In addition to initial suggestions by students, I brought an array of possible books to class for potential reading by students over a vacation period. The bibliography kept expanding with *Walking Down the Street* (Treitel, 2000) chosen for the Author's Forum. Give and take between students and author was animated, particularly as she described having dealt with her own learning dysfunction and the support and lack of support she encountered on the way to recognizing her ability to write. It has been said that life is like going up a down escalator. If you do not continually try to go higher, you actually move lower. To grow spiritually we need to strive upward. Physician Carlos Werter speaks of the healing pyramid, also recognizing the importance of reaching higher spiritual levels (Werter, 1999). Treitel's book includes a poem entitled "Growing" (p. 173):

A person's
growth
is applied
in layers.

Each
new insight

has to be
measured,
adjusted
and tried on.

Layering
ourselves
is dressing
our soul.

– M. T. Treitel

For many, 9/11 was the new impetus for spiritual growth. Sales of spirituality books after 9/11 sky rocketed. *The New York Times* reported that scientists are trying to find reasons for the new broad interest in religion (Lee, 2002).

There has been a proliferation of spirituality-related 9/11 Web resources. Dr. Johnson's poem opened the 9/11 section of headcleaners.com. Excerpts follow: "May our actions be motivated more by humanity and thought than by anger and fear . . . May we all keep in mind that it makes no sense to become what we hate. May we all keep in mind that one day we all die and that *how* we live until then is probably more important than how long we live or how leisurely."

Emmy award-winning engineer Mark Schubin expressed similar sentiments about hate in his post-9/11 Web-based Schubin Chronicles, which earned international circulation. However, in addition to providing daily updates from a New Yorker's perspective, he added positive activities to do, ranging from unique supermarkets to visit to books for reading to each other (Schubin, 2001-2002). Dr. Werter recognizes the deleterious impact of complaining and suggests that in the midst of complaints by others we remain silent rather than adding further negativity to the atmosphere (Werter, 1999).

When asked to speak at a community event, I initially called the talk "An Upbeat Look at Revenge." While many thought of revenge immediately after 9/11, time has begun to steer responses in different directions. I prepared to ask the audience to consider seven lessons that we can learn from the letters of revenge and related actions that could be taken.

R–Reconsider the benefit-harm ratio before reacting. Refresh your memory about a scenario that benefited from reflection. With your eyes closed, imagine a current dilemma or expected anxiety; picture yourself above it for an objective view.

E–Extrapolate positively toward the future. Separate the trivialities from what will still be important twenty years from now. Think of something that you can let go, including a grudge.

V–Value what you do have. Consider creating a gratitude booklet.

E–Engage in constructive activities. Do something productive.

N–Nurture your own spiritual sense. When you focus on one thing, you are less likely to see another.

G–Gladden the lives of yourself and others. Consider who you like to be around and why. Try to emulate a role model of your choice.

E–Enlighten others with your own spirituality. Teach. Share. Learn together.

As my spirituality efforts matured, I became involved in the expanding science and religion field, attending a training workshop and seminars, earning honorable mention for designing a course, co-writing a 9/11 article (Greenberg & Heltzel, 2002) and speaking about it at a scholar's event. Post-9/11 articles initially reported an increasing movement toward faith. In October 2001, *Newsweek* magazine noted as an example that St. Patrick's Cathedral in New York City had increased daily masses to six. The same issue reported that 400 couples in Houston, Texas had withdrawn their divorce papers because the event taught them the importance of family values. Months later, a tapering off in the increased participation in formal worship attendance was noted. Yet, *U.S. News & World Report,* in May 2002 had a cover story, "Faith in America," that brought responses into July on the importance of spirituality at this time.

How did people cope with 9/11 and how are they continuing to cope thereafter? Although some remained "glued to the television" and may be the purchasers of the many books that are primarily photo collections, others sought spirituality. Even the photographic volumes included that element. *Brotherhood*, which focuses on firefighters, begins with a photo of Mayor Rudy Giuliani with the palms of his hands together in a traditional prayer position and ends with a firefighter's prayer. *Nation*, which was the bestseller of the 9/11 books, includes a photo of a person kneeling in a field almost a continent away where wooden crosses had been erected to represent those lives lost on September 11. Is the post-event patriotism a type of spiritual occupation? A photo in an occupational therapy publication captioned a photograph showing "God Bless America" graffiti as patriotic (Diffendal, 2002). By the one-year anniversary more than 150 books related to 9/11 had been published (Minzesheimer, 2002).

I was fortunate in being able to connect with students at Stuyvesant High School, which served as the triage center on September 11th, 2001. Students suggested that an epidemiological study follow them over time to assess the environmental impact of September 11. Among the philanthropic gifts to the school was $25,000 worth of large live plants to handle the excess carbon monoxide in the air. As evidence of the mandate to carry on, student "plant parents" were designated to take care of the plants, which are everywhere. Stuyvesant teacher Roz Bierig received the Teacher Who Made a Difference award from the Revson Foundation. She coordinated the Bioethics Symposium in which I participated shortly after students were allowed back in the school, just two months following 9/11. Panelists ranged from a neurologist to a Catholic priest, considering what it means to be human in an environment increasingly dominated by modern technology. It was a humbling experience. The auditorium was packed with students who chose to return after school to ponder the questions of life and death and the advance of health through technology. These are the same students who only months before had watched people jump from the towers of the World Trade Center holding hands. The priest told how he was stopped on the way to the school, as clergy were needed at the temporary morgue set up at Ground Zero.

We can learn humility and reverence even from what appear to be ordinary inanimate objects. Can we see a new perspective when we know that the dump truck in Photo 7 is carrying remains from Ground Zero as it passes under the Tribeca pedestrian bridge leading to Stuyvesant High School? Imagine all the occupations involved in the "clean-up." From the truck drivers to those sorting through the rubble in Staten Island, there was a new spiritual dimension to their tasks. At the ceremony marking the close of the sorting site, the director was asked what kept them going for ten months. He calmly answered, "the families." The motivation was that, perhaps, they could find some body part, some memento that could provide solace to the families.

Seeing a sign at Ground Zero (Photo 8) that clearly delineated a separation made me wonder about how we each make separations between what we consider to be spiritual and what is not. The sign implies potential contamination. What is the contaminant to our own spiritual

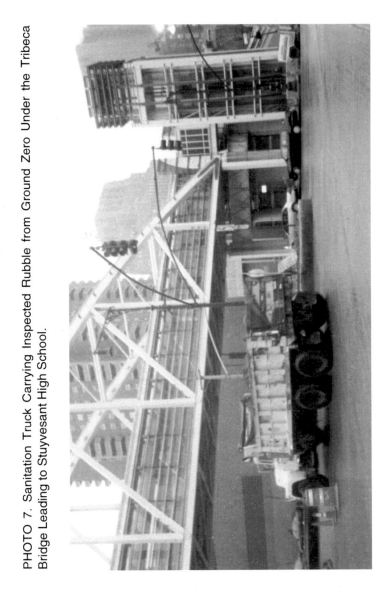

PHOTO 7. Sanitation Truck Carrying Inspected Rubble from Ground Zero Under the Tribeca Bridge Leading to Stuyvesant High School.

Photo by Naomi Greenberg. Used by permission.

PHOTO 8. A Sign of the Times at Ground Zero.

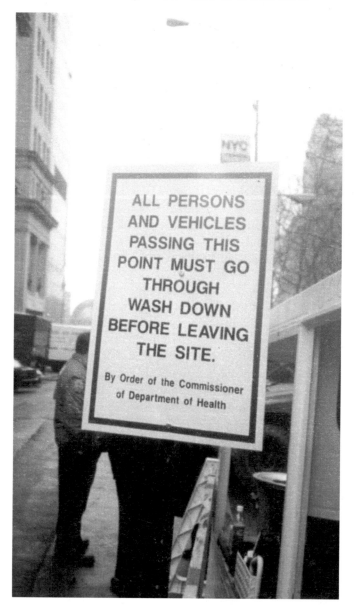

Photo by Naomi Greenberg. Used by permission.

growth? A washing station hidden among the memorabilia (Photo 9) was almost a surprise discovery. Was it for convenience, to use after potential environmental exposure or for something more? Many religions designate water for purification, even encouraging cleansing before prayer and after visiting a grave or cemetery.

The landscape of New York is altered. The Twin Towers are gone. The air quality changed. The transportation system was affected, and lives are more complicated. When several things are taken out of whack, everything else feels the impact. All things in our environment are dependent on everything else. In a changing situation, many turn toward spirituality for healing. Some sought outlets of expression in projects such as planting flowers. The bouquet of flowers placed in the fence near Ground Zero (Photo 10) may be a similar expression of spirituality, the spontaneous kind. Graduate students from Manhattan's residential International House raked leaves and planted 2,000 memorial daffodil buds in Sakura Park on the Upper West Side. As an activity of their local environmental activism group, here was a small way they could honor the loss of life through active gardening and environmental care taking. The huge increase in ferry service from downtown Manhattan to New Jersey as a substitute for the destroyed train services below the World Trade Center provided commuters with the beauty of experiencing the open-air environment while riding on top of the Hudson River instead of underground. When I took the new Hoboken ferry, I was reminded of traveling on older and larger ones as they moved through ice chunks during my childhood. Life goes on.

The Disaster Spiritual Care Committee of the American Red Cross in Greater New York convened a day-long conference in June 2002 to help more than 900 religious leaders understand the scope of the post-9/11 problems and provide strategies to help cope with them. Articles about the conference, "The Life Cycle of a Disaster: Understanding the Impact of the 9/11 Terrorist Attacks on Faith Communities and Their Leaders," emphasized the importance of healing the healers with a focus on religious leaders' "compassion fatigue" following 9/11. Described as one of the largest interfaith gatherings in New York City history, the conference reported that the numbers of people turning to religious leaders for consultation is increasing rather than decreasing. Participants were warned that the impact of September 11 will be long-term, to be measured in years. The therapy suggested for the clergy is what they are suggesting to others: exercise, laughing, taking a vacation and talking with a member of a faith group.

PHOTO 9. This Washing Station Is Among the Temporary Additions Outside Saint Paul's Church.

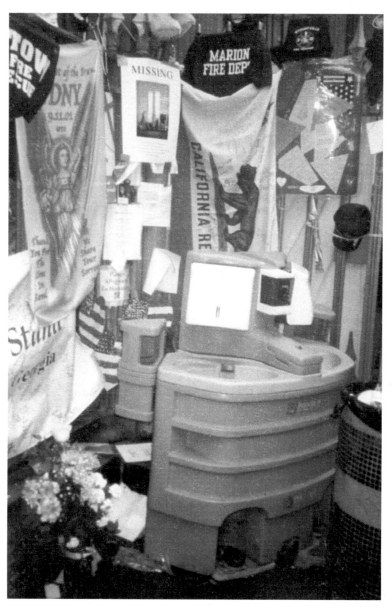

Photo by Naomi Greenberg. Used by permission.

PHOTO 10. Flowers Placed in a Fence of a New York City Street Near Battery Park. Spiritual Spontaneity?

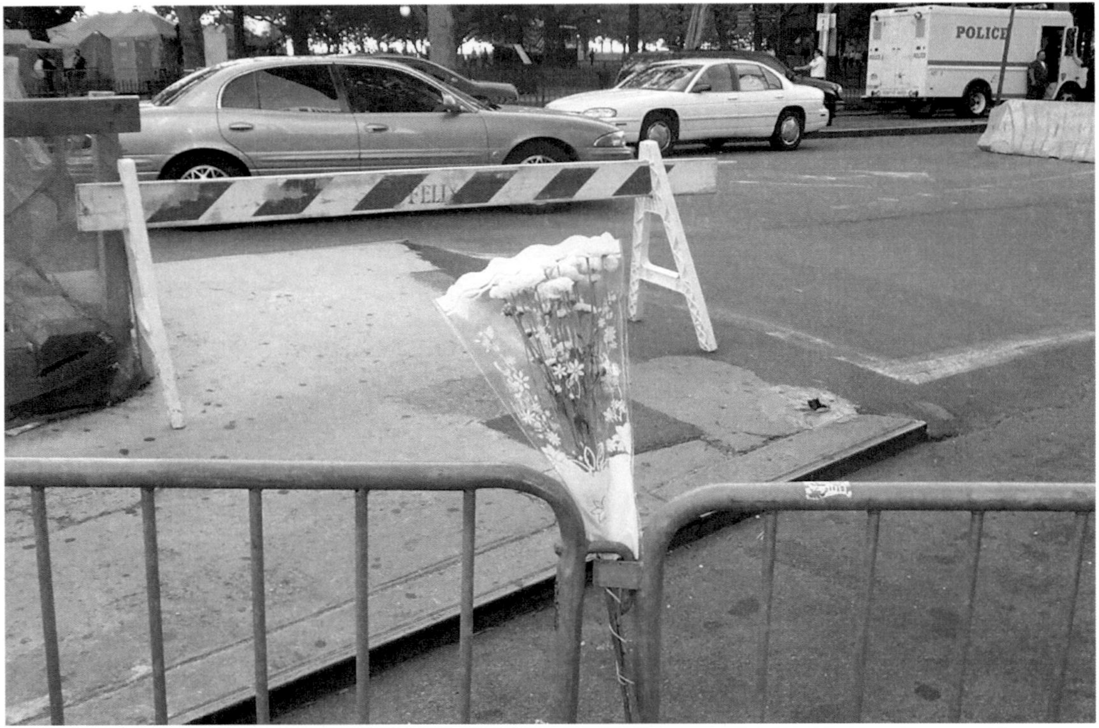

Photo by Pat Precin. Used by permission.

Occupational therapy practitioners could easily add to that list. Hands-on is a term that has been used with regard to faith healing. I once completed a workshop in therapeutic touch where I learned that touch can improve mood and strengthen the immune system. It is therefore a necessity for a healthy life. Ask why volunteers did what they did after 9/11 and you may hear, "to lend a helping hand." Hands can be representative of many helpful approaches including spirituality. Among the many items sent to Ground Zero was a display of handprints from a school in Massachusetts (Photo 11).

I was privileged to see a fantastic new Hands exhibit at the Israel Museum in Jerusalem. The exhibit poster showed an array of pairs of hands coming together in a circle in the sand, a simple yet sensual and spiritual statement. The brochure opened with the fact that depictions of hands have been considered protective since early cave history. Interactive computer stations enabled visitors to select from playful hands, productive hands, interpretive hands, creative hands, spiritual hands and more. Links that ranged from ancient sculpture to string figures brought art work and learning into focus. Based in the Youth Wing, the exhibit gave children and adults the opportunity to get involved with a multiplicity of experiences related to hands. Activities and displays included such diverse opportunities as curtained stereognosis set-ups, prostheses, puppets of all types, textured surfaces ranging from rubberized projections to marble balls, hands holding long braids to the side, hands painted as animals and sports figures, hands used to crawl through tunnels, cranked robots, molded hand-shaped chairs, a wooden hand large enough to climb into and giant hand projections that moved when a person approached. Many of the exhibits could be duplicated elsewhere in a simpler fashion to bring smiles and interaction in a post-9/11 atmosphere.

What is on the horizon? Lectures and programs already scheduled include "Spirituality in the Face of Adversity" and "Building Safe Communities: Coping with Uncertainty and Violence." As early as six months after 9/11, several movies and documentaries on the subject were already being prepared. Some said that was too soon. With the impact on the economy, articles on Web sites appeared on topics such as practical strategies for understanding and coping with the challenges of losing a job as a result of the terrorist attack of 9/11. As the first anniversary approached, there was renewed interest and coverage on many levels. Frontline on public television featured clergy and lay reflections on God. Public radio offered perspectives from around the world associated with the phrase "that sad September." The Boulder [Colorado]

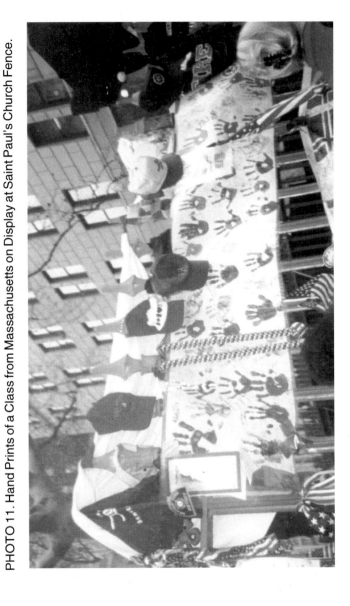

PHOTO 11. Hand Prints of a Class from Massachusetts on Display at Saint Paul's Church Fence.

Photo by Naomi Greenberg. Used by permission.

News pointed out that people differ as to how 9/11 changed them. LaGuardia Community College scheduled its first day of classes for September 11, 2002, so that there could be a special commemorative program with a publication featuring feelings then and now.

In conjunction with the movement toward fostering spirituality with health came a January 2002 call for proposals for "Scientific Research on Unlimited Love: Altruism, Compassion and Service." Remembering my efforts with The Random Acts of Kindness Foundation and my use of the concepts at a 6:30 a.m. stress management session for the security staff at LaGuardia Community College, I began to think of a new project. I found a sociologist to work with me on the theme and submitted a proposal. A monthly column on unlimited love now appears in *Research News and Opportunities in Science and Theology* along with a column on "Faith in Action."

Although not the same meaning as *New York* magazine's "Love After 9/11," the report of increasing interest in marriage and decreasing emphasis on a potential spouse having a good job could be recognition of a more spiritual direction. Reports of what may be considered more positive values is in keeping with the altruism, compassion and service seen post- 9/11. Articles published immediately thereafter, at the 3-month postmark, the 6-month postmark and for the first Independence Day after the event included diverse examples of unlimited love. Little did we know what kind of a world we would be facing post-September 2001. People became more aware of being surrounded by "In God We Trust," "One nation under God," and the music of Irving Berlin's "God Bless America." The September 2002 issue of *Ladies' Home Journal* reported the results of a poll indicating that 45% of readers are "praying more" since 9/11/01.

Is there a place for spirituality in occupational therapy? Perhaps, after 9/11, we may need it as much, if not more, for ourselves as for our clients. It has been said that there is less burnout among truly spiritual people because they can share the joy and sadness of others without expecting anything in return. Like the physicians that Rachel Remen has to deprogram from their medical training, many of us were taught in our occupational therapy training to remain objective and depersonalized. Yet, if we consider a client-centered approach and the client is reaching for spiritual engagement, should we always only refer elsewhere? Articles related to spirituality in the occupational therapy literature cover topics ranging from the need to teach potential therapists spirituality, to avoiding negative interactions, to actual therapeutic use of direct spiritual activities such as prayer.

In *The Spiritual Realm of Occupational Therapy* (Gourley, 2001, pgs. 13-14), the focus is on occupational therapist Liz Allen, a part-time chaplain. "Although most OTs do not realize it, they are ministers to the soul." The American Occupational Therapy Association has designed new "Tips for Living" sheets. One is on gardening. Occupational therapy practitioners in mental health have used horticultural therapy effectively to meet both long-term and short-term goals. Although the tip sheet addresses only physical issues, many people participated after 9/11 in faith-based gardening efforts. Planting flower bulbs was at the same time a physical outlet and a spiritual opportunity to project renewed growth and beauty on the horizon.

In a series of workshops funded by the Templeton Foundation, St. Vincent's Hospital, the site that received the 9/11 injured, recognized the need for spiritual involvement of health professionals. When a client is seeking solace and a listening ear, the situation may not be able to wait for clergy, or the words may be directed intentionally toward the health professional. Each workshop session began with an actual case presentation related to the theme for that week and was followed by a debate by invited representatives of two religions. An example for the theme, "Forgiveness and the Care of the Patient," focused on a man who, anticipating death, wondered whether he should share his past indiscretions with his wife. The debate considered theological views, but focused on issues such as from whom was the patient seeking forgiveness (from God, from the wife, or from the health professional approached), the role of the health professional to whom he reveals his concern, the possibility that the wife may already know and should be able to choose whether or not she wants the issue openly raised and more.

In bioethics courses, I teach about autonomy, and the American Occupational Therapy Association Code of Ethics and Guidelines holds that therapists should not discriminate in their delivery of treatment. But that does not preclude a spiritual therapeutic use of self on behalf of a client where appropriate. What does Spiritual Spontaneity have to do with occupational therapy? It can be the motivation to work toward therapeutic goals. It can be the foundation for promoting socialization and positive interactions. Each of the occupations in Table 3 can be expanded to activities and projects. For example, "thank" can be the impetus for a gratitude notebook, a poster display or a theme for a discussion group.

When scheduled to conduct evaluations at a nursing home one month after 9/11 and finding that there were few patients available for them, I used the opportunity to connect with residents for an informal survey. Having been a full-time nursing home consultant at ten facilities, I was used to dealing with their concerns. In this new era, I was amazed at the responses! The consensus was an almost unanimous, "Appreciate Life." Is it possible that my own Spiritual Spontaneity reflected back to theirs? I first tested my theory and Spiritual Spontaneity Scale: Evaluating Our Own 9-11 (Table 4) at a charity luncheon for which I was the invited guest speaker. For a subsequent group I developed Spiritual Spontaneity Steps: Practicing and Perfecting Our Own 9-11 (Table 5). Both are effective for goal progression and selecting areas to address.

So what is the message? Perhaps it is that we need to find our own message while allowing others to do so as well. Reflection and time to ponder can help answer the questions: "What is this meant to teach me? Where is my role? How should I try to grow from this experience?" A sage, the Baal Shem Tov, offered ancient wisdom: There are three things needed for growth: humility, discrimination and conciliation.

Like so many others since 9/11, I have been devouring audiotapes, lectures, readings and more. Several teach ways to strive toward spiritual greatness. Lists include simple approaches such as offering a smile or doing an unannounced kindness, particularly appreciating the value of each and every individual and making a contribution to society. Perhaps, through such preparation, we will be able to further develop the spiritual spontaneity to deal with the unexpected, the unanticipated,

TABLE 3. Occupations for Spiritual Spontaneity

1	S	smile	1	S	simplify
2	P	ponder	2	P	praise
3	I	imagine	3	O	optimize
4	R	reflect	4	N	network
5	I	identify	5	T	transcend
6	T	talk	6	A	accept
7	U	unify	7	N	notice
8	A	aspire	8	E	elevate
9	L	love	9	I	inspire
			10	T	thank
			11	Y	yearn

when it arrives. Years ago I attended a workshop to prepare for my first spiritual outreach trip to the former Soviet Union when it was still illegal. One lesson remains with me. We travel through time as though a train on a track. At each station of the year, whether holidays or quarterly milestones we pick up something useful and continue the journey. As this remarkable year drew to a close, the media was again teeming with 9/11-related content. May we be blessed with the ability to select that which will help us to grow spiritually. Thanks for accompanying me on the journey.

At the 9/11 anniversary event at LaGuardia Community College the college president spoke of hope and clear beginnings. My Spiritual Spontaneity reflections were read from the stage by a student highlighted by a dim light in a darkened room with two towers of smoke rising behind him against a city view. The audience spontaneously began to rhythmically move arms overhead as four international students did so to the words of "Heal the World." The finale was productive activity as we formed a procession to the cobblestone courtyard where each member of the college community present had an opportunity to add a spade of dirt to a newly planted tree. The theme was that the day should be remembered for the positive changes it brought in our relationships with others.

Just as in the Lamaze method through which I prepared through conditioning for the pangs of childbirth, perhaps we can condition ourselves to be ready with spiritual solutions for situations as they arise. In a session entitled "Yearning for Perfection," Aaron Raaps described the moon as building toward its peak each month only to wane again. Although we do not expect to achieve lasting perfection, it is the yearning that matters. If we keep the spiritual messages we choose upon our hearts, then when our heart breaks, as it has with terrorist attacks, at that one right moment, the spiritual message can fall into the heart. We will then, hopefully, be ready to share our spirituality with others as it continues to provide solace for us.

CONCLUSION

Drawing from a variety of sources, the question of spirituality has been examined in light of the lessons of 9/11. Highlights of recent findings were culled from four key areas, post-September 11 reports, the proliferating science and religion movement, the vast array of spirituality literature, and the awakening within occupational therapy. On an international and national level, occupational therapy had begun to recognize the importance of considering spirituality in assessment and treatment planning. Perhaps this new awakening will help occupational therapy practitioners to realize that it is all right to consider their own spirituality as they address that of their clients.

ISSUES FOR FUTURE CONSIDERATION

- Collect inspirational stories of lessons learned as a result of 9/11.
- Contrast original reactions to 9/11 with subsequent spiritual perspectives.
- Examine "therapeutic use of self" from a spiritual perspective.
- Evaluate effectiveness of Steps toward promoting spiritual growth.
- Identify already used activities that could be adapted to introduce a spiritual dimension.
- Interview clients and families regarding spiritual occupations.
- Survey occupational therapy practitioners as to their own post-9/11 spiritual growth.
- Test the Spiritual Spontaneity Scale on two specific populations.

ACKNOWLEDGMENTS

Appreciation is extended to the occupational therapy practitioners who participated in the activities described above, to those who offered suggestions–particularly librarian Louise Fluk, and to *Research News*–and my co-author Peter Heltzel for permission to include sections of *Where Is God in the Rubble?*

REFERENCES

Adahan, M. (1995). *Calm down: Taking control of your life* (p. 230). Southfield, Michigan: Targum Press.

American Occupational Therapy Association, Inc. (2002). *Occupational therapy practice framework domain and process* (p. 63 of draft).

American Psychiatric Association. (2000). *Diagnostic and statistical manual of mental disorders (text revision)*. Washington, DC: Author.

Band of Angels Website: (http://www.bandofangels.net.inspfaith.htm). Cited in Bits and Pieces.

Cottrell, R. F. (2001). Resilience reaffirmed. *Advance for Occupational Therapy Practitioners, 17,* (22) 4.

Davis, J. (July 2001). *Can prayer heal?* Website: (http://www.content.health.msn.com/)

Diffendal, J. (2002, July 15). Remembering and rebuilding New York: OTs recount their efforts in 9/11 recovery. *Advance for Occupational Therapy Practitioners, 39 & 44.*

Emerson, G., Howell, R., & Scott, J. (Introduction). (2002). *Portraits: 9/11/01.* New York: Times Books/Henry Holt and Company.

Gourley, M. (Ed.). (2001). The spiritual realm of occupational therapy. *OT Practice, 6*(8), 13-14.

Graham, B. (2002, May/June). Making peace with fear. *AARP, 58.*

Greenberg, N. (2001). *Incorporating spirituality into science content.* Presentation at New York State Occupational Therapy Association Annual Conference, Albany.

Greenberg, N. & Heltzel, P. (2002, February). Where Is God in the Rubble? *Research News.*

Greenberg, N. & Lewis, B. (1995). Using Holiday Traditions to Achieve Therapeutic Goals. *Advance for Occupational Therapists, 11*(50), 11.

Hirshfield, N. (2002, April). The force of a woman. *Oprah Magazine.* 22.

Hume, C. A. (1998). Spiritual care: The unrecognized dimension of occupational therapy? Presentation at International Congress of the World Federation of Occupational Therapists, Montreal.

Jacobs, K., & Jacobs, L. (2001). *Quick reference dictionary for occupational therapy.* Thoroughfare, NJ: Slack, 180.

Keith, K. M. (2002). *Anyway: The paradoxical commandments: Finding personal meaning in a crazy world.* New York: G.P. Putnam's Sons.

King, D. E. (2000). *Faith, spirituality, and medicine: Toward the making of the healing practitioner.* New York: Haworth Pastoral Press.

Lee, F. R. (2002, Aug 24). The secular society gets religion. *New York Times Arts & Ideas/Cultural Desk,* B7.

Levy, A. (2002, Feb.) Love after 9/11. *New York Magazine,* 18-20.

Lohr, S. (2001, November 18) Gearhead nation: A time out for technophilia. *The New York Times,* Sect. 4, 4.

Low, A. (1997). *Mental health through will training.* Reprinted edition. Winnetka, IL: Willett Publishers.

Mayers, C. A. (1998). *'Spiritual' well-being: Is this part of our role?* Presentation at International Congress of the World Federation of Occupational Therapists, Montreal.

Meador, K. (2002). Being well, living well and dying well. *Research News and Opportunities in Science and Religion, 2*(11/12), 7.

Michaud, E. (2002, May). Bouncing back. *Prevention.*

Minzesheimer, B. (2002, August 13). Sept. 11 inspires record number of 'event' books. *USA Today.*

North, C. S., Pfefferbaum, B. (2002, August 7). Research in the mental health effects of terrorism. *Journal of the American Medical Association: 288*(5), 633-636.

Otterness, T. (2001). *Lighten up: Art with a sense of humor.* Exhibit at De Cordova Museum Sculpture Park, Lincoln, Massachusetts.

Puchalsky, C. (2002). The spirit of medicine in research news and opportunities. *Science and Religion,* 2(11/12), 5-6.

Quotes Happiness 019.0. Webpage: <http://enchanted/>attic.net/QuotesHappiness.html

Remen, R. N. (1997). *Kitchen Table Wisdom: Stories That Heal.* New York: T. Berkely.

Remen, R. N. (2000). *My Grandfather's Blessings.* New York: Penguin Putnam.

Remen, R. N. (2001, Fall). Recovering doctors. *City Spirit.*

Rosenfeld, M. S. (2000, Jan.17). Spiritual agent modalities for occupational therapy practice. *OT Practice, 17-21.*

Rosenfeld, M. S. (2001, June 18). Spiritual context for care. *OT Practice,* 6(11), 19-20 & 22-25.

Schlenger, W. E., Cadell, J. M., Ebert, L., Jordan, B. K., Dennis, J. M., Fairbank, J. A. et al. (2002). Psychological reactions to terrorist attacks: Findings from the national study of Americans' reactions to September 11. *Journal of the American Medical Association 288*: 581-588.

Schubin, M. (2001-2002). *The Schubin chronicles.* (www.symes.tv/schubin_chronicles. htm)

Sheler, J. L., Curry, A., Kulman, L., & Gilgoff, D. (2002, May 6). Faith in America. *US News & World Report.*

Sorensen, J. (1998). How metaphysics interacts with OT. In *Advance for Occupational Therapy Practitioners 14,* (22), 6.

Steinsaltz, A. (2001). *Simple words: Thinking about what really matters in life.* New York: Touchstone Books. Simon and Schuster, 54-55.

Swanson, A. (2002). Dealing with the loss of a loved one through celebration. *Research News and Opportunities in Science and Theology,* 2(11/12,) 24.

Taylor, E., Mitchell, J., Kenan, S., & Tucker, R. (2000). Attitudes of occupational therapists toward spirituality in practice. *American Journal of Occupational Therapy,* 54(4), 421-426.

Thibodaux, L. R. (1998). Acknowledging the spiritual visions in treatment. Presentation at International Congress of the World Federation of Occupational Therapists, Montreal.

Treitel, M. F. (2000). *Walking down the street: Observations along the road of life, 173.* Brooklyn, NY: Shaar Press/Mesorah Publications.

Tsai, E. (2002). The worlds of Tom Otterness. In T. Otterness (Ed.), *Tom Otterness: Free money and other fairy tales* (4). New York: Marlborough.

Viereck, G. S. (1929, October 26) What life means to Einstein. *The Saturday Evening Post.*

Wells, S. & Maher, J. (September 28, 2001). AP photographer stands by his work. (9News.com/newsroom/13294.html)

Weiss, F., & Cecala, T. (2002, Winter). Website: (http://www.holisticnetworker.com/ editorial/bethechange.html)

Werter, C. (1999). *Who do you think you are?* New York: Bantam.

TABLE 4. Spiritual Spontaneity Scale Testing Your Own 9-11

What one **action** most represents spiritual spontaneity to you? _____

Instructions:
Please check off your first response, realizing that you need at least one in each column to have FON/fun.

Do you consider yourself to be a spiritual person? yes _____ no _____ maybe _____

How long does it take you to gain a spiritual perspective of an event or remark?
minutes_____ hours _____ days _____ weeks _____ months _____ years _____

	frequently/ F	occasionally/ O	almost never N
Part I			
1. How often do you **smile**?	____	____	____
2. Do you **ponder** how your words might impact on the listener?	____	____	____
3. Are you able to **imagine** a positive perspective no matter what the situation?	____	____	____
4. Do you **reflect** on your spiritual responses once they have occurred?	____	____	____
5. Are you able to **identify** with a person's grief or joy?	____	____	____
6. Do you **talk** positively about other people?	____	____	____
7. Can you think of a spiritual way to **unify** individuals and or groups?	____	____	____
8. Do you **aspire** to greater levels of spirituality?	____	____	____
9. Are you able to grant or consider unconditional **love**?	____	____	____

Scoring: frequently = 1 point, occasionally = 1/2 point, almost never = 0 points

Part I perfect score = 9   Your score _____

Part II			
1. Can you **simplify** your life to incorporate spiritual connections and growth?	____	____	____
2. Does **praise** for a person, item or experience come easily for you?	____	____	____
3. Do you **optimize** your spiritual opportunities?	____	____	____
4. Do you choose to **network** with people who think positively or spiritually?	____	____	____
5. Can you **transcend** an initial response or immediate concern toward a better future?	____	____	____
6. Can you **accept** things over which you have no control?	____	____	____
7. Do you **notice** the best in people and events?	____	____	____
8. How often do you try to **elevate** another person's status through respect?	____	____	____
9. Do you **inspire** others through words, deeds or actions?	____	____	____
10. Do you **thank** people with sincerity and/or keep your own gratitude book?	____	____	____
11. Do you **yearn** for perfection?	____	____	____

Part II Scoring: frequently = 1 point, occasionally = 1/2 point, almost never = 0

Part II perfect score = 11   Your score _____

	Part I	Part II
Perfect Score	9	- 11
Your Score	____	- ____

Congratulations! Wherever you are on the scale, you're well on your way toward the unreachable perfection of
9-11.

Spiritual = 9. Spontaneity = 11. Spiritual Spontaneity = 9-11. Keep yearning and learning!

TABLE 5. Spiritual Spontaneity Steps:
Practicing Your Own 9-11

Nine Days to Spiritual Spontaneity

January 9th. Between 9p.m. tonight and 11p.m. tomorrow night I will try to
smile to at least one more person (among those I know and those I don't know) than I usually do.

February 9th. Between 9p.m. tonight and 11p.m. tomorrow night I will try to
ponder the potential impact of my words on at least two people before speaking.

March 9th. Between 9p.m. tonight and 11p.m. tomorrow night I will try to
imagine a positive scenario for three situations I am facing.

April 9th. Between 9p.m. tonight and 11p.m. tomorrow night I will try to
unify people I know by spending at least four minutes planning a way to do so.

May 9th. Between 9p.m. tonight and 11p.m. tomorrow night I will try to
individualize my communication with five people toward their goals rather than my designs for them.

June 6th. Between 9p.m. tonight and 11p.m. tomorrow night I will try to
talk only positively about others for six hours.

July 9th. Between 9p.m. tonight and 11p.m. tomorrow night I will try to
reflect on seven of my responses and interactions toward a more spiritual way for next time.

August 8th. Between 9p.m. tonight and 11p.m. tomorrow night I will try to
aspire to greater levels of spiritually in eight areas of my life.

September 9th. Between 9p.m. tonight and 11p.m. tomorrow night I will try to
love for nine minutes without expecting anything in return.

Eleven Days to Spiritual Spontaneity

January 11th. Between 9p.m. tonight and 11p.m. tomorrow night I will try to
simplify my life in at least one way to allow for spiritual growth.

February 11th. Between 9p.m. tonight and 11p.m. tomorrow night I will try to
praise at least two persons, items or experiences.

March 11th. Between 9p.m. tonight and 11p.m. tomorrow night I will try to
optimize my spiritual opportunities by looking for three everyday miracles.

April 11th. Between 9p.m. tonight and 11p.m. tomorrow night I will try to
network with people toward a spiritual project. (e.g., charity fund raiser, visitors for sick, etc.)

May 11th. Between 9p.m. tonight and 11p.m. tomorrow night I will try to
transend five remarks or observations and my reactions to them toward more spiritual responses.

June 11th. Between 9p.m. tonight and 11p.m. tomorrow night I will try to
accept things that I have no control over for a minimum of six minutes.

July 11th. Between 9p.m. tonight and 11p.m. tomorrow night I will try to
notice the best in four people or events.

August 11th. Between 9p.m. tonight and 11p.m. tomorrow night I will try to
elevate another person's status by recognizing eight positive attributes.

September 11th. Between 9p.m. tonight and 11p.m. tomorrow night I will try to
inspire nine people including myself.

October 11th. Between 9p.m. tonight and 11p.m. tomorrow night I will try to
thank ten people and/or write ten things for which I am grateful.

November 11th. Between 9p.m. tonight and 11p.m. tomorrow night I will try to
yearn for perfection for at least eleven minutes without focusing on imperfection.

Index

Surviving 9/11

Impact and Experiences
of Occupational Therapy Practitioners

___ in softbound at $18.71 (regularly $24.95) (ISBN: 0-7890-2067-X)
___ in hardbound at $29.96 (regularly $39.95) (ISBN: 0-7890-2066-1)

COST OF BOOKS ___

Outside USA/ Canada/
Mexico: Add 20%. ___

POSTAGE & HANDLING ___

US: $4.00 for first book & $1.50
for each additional book
Outside US: $5.00 for first book
& $2.00 for each additional book.

SUBTOTAL ___

In Canada: add 7% GST. ___

STATE TAX ___

CA, IL, IN, MIN, NY, OH, & SD residents
please add appropriate local sales tax.

FINAL TOTAL ___

If paying in Canadian funds, convert
using the current exchange rate,
UNESCO coupons welcome.

❏ **BILL ME LATER:**

Bill-me option is good on US/Canada/
Mexico orders only; not good to jobbers,
wholesalers, or subscription agencies.

❏ **Signature** ___

❏ **Payment Enclosed: $** ___

❏ **PLEASE CHARGE TO MY CREDIT CARD:**

❏ Visa ❏ MasterCard ❏ AmEx ❏ Discover
❏ Diner's Club ❏ Eurocard ❏ JCB

Account # ___

Exp Date ___

Signature ___

*(Prices in US dollars and subject to
change without notice.)*

PLEASE PRINT ALL INFORMATION OR ATTACH YOUR BUSINESS CARD
Name
Address
City   State/Province   Zip/Postal Code
Country
Tel   Fax
E-Mail

May we use your e-mail address for confirmations and other types of information? ❏Yes ❏ No
We appreciate receiving your e-mail address. Haworth would like to e-mail special discount
offers to you, as a preferred customer. **We will never share, rent, or exchange your e-mail
address.** We regard such actions as an invasion of your privacy.

Order From Your Local Bookstore or Directly From
The Haworth Press, Inc.
10 Alice Street, Binghamton, New York 13904-1580 • USA
Call Our toll-free number (1-800-429-6784) / Outside US/Canada: (607) 722-5857
Fax: 1-800-895-0582 / Outside US/Canada: (607) 771-0012
E-Mail your order to us: Orders@haworthpress.com

Please Photocopy this form for your personal use.
www.HaworthPress.com

BOF04